THYROID GUARDIAN OF HEALTH

PHILIP G. YOUNG MD

Printed in Victoria, Canada

National Library of Canada Cataloguing in Publication

Young, Philip G. (Philip Gibbs)
 Thyroid, guardian of health / Philip G. Young.
Includes bibliographical references.
ISBN 1-55369-613-1
 1. Hypothyroidism--Popular works. I. Title.
RC657.Y69 2002   616.4'44   C2002-902520-6

TRAFFORD

This book was published *on-demand* in cooperation with Trafford Publishing.
On-demand publishing is a unique process and service of making a book available for retail sale to the public taking advantage of on-demand manufacturing and Internet marketing.
On-demand publishing includes promotions, retail sales, manufacturing, order fulfilment, accounting and collecting royalties on behalf of the author.

Suite 6E, 2333 Government St., Victoria, B.C. V8T 4P4, CANADA
Phone   250-383-6864   Toll-free 1-888-232-4444 (Canada & US)
Fax   250-383-6804   E-mail   sales@trafford.com
Web site   www.trafford.com TRAFFORD PUBLISHING IS A DIVISION OF TRAFFORD HOLDINGS LTD.
Trafford Catalogue #02-0426   www.trafford.com/robots/02-0426.html

10   9   8   7   6   5   4   3   2   1

DISCLAIMER

The information in this book is based on an interest in the thyroid gland for over twenty years and includes extensive reading of the medical literature and working with individuals with thyroid problems over this period. This book is intended to inform the public on the necessity of adequate thyroid function in good health and is not intended as replacement of sound medical advice from a physician. Sharing the information in this book with the attending physician is desirable. Application of the information and recommendations given within are undertaken at the individuals own risk.

All the recommendations contained herein are made without guarantee on the part of the author, the publisher, their agents, or employees. The author and the publisher disclaim all liability in connection with the use of the information presented in this book.

INDEX

Preface

A young woman wastes away under the onslaught of tuberculosis; another young woman weeps because she has been unable to bear a child; a man, still in his prime, clutches his chest as an unexpected heart attack cuts him down; a child squirms day after day in the classroom, his head a muddle, unable to grasp the latest lesson; a lady is depressed for no seeming reason---what do these individuals share in common? Each may be suffering from undiagnosed hypothyroidism. Proper treatment with thyroid replacement therapy could change these lives. The young woman with tuberculosis could rise out of her sick bed. The other woman could be cradling a baby. The man could be attending the latest business meeting. The child could be mastering his lessons. And the depressed lady could find joy in living again. Why isn't this happening? Why are so many preventable tragedies like these still taking place? To find the answer let's begin with the thyroid story.

The thyroid is a gland that lies in the front of the neck. Early anatomists gave it its name from a Latin word meaning shield, perhaps due to its shape. It is the body's shield against a host of infirmities because thyroid hormone controls metabolism. In layman's terms, it controls the energy available to the body, which means it controls the energy the body uses to complete all its tasks. If not enough energy is available, some of the functions of the body are going to be shortchanged. The body may not have enough energy to fight infection. The body may not have the energy for reproductive functions to occur normally or the body may not have the energy to repair itself, and the arteries may harden until a heart stops beating or a stroke occurs. The brain may not have the energy it needs to function, so it may be hard to learn lessons in school or it may be difficult to control emotions.

Although thyroid controls metabolism, it teams up with other hormones and other processes to see that the body produces the energy it needs. Metabolism also depends upon the body's fuel intake, the quality and quantity of food that is eaten. So all the digestive enzymes form part of the energy production team of the body. The storage and transport of that fuel to the cells is controlled by the adrenal hormones, the glucocorticoids. The handling of body's main fuel, glucose, is actually impacted by a host of other hormones such as insulin. So the energy output of the body depends on the triad of fuel, transport and the regulation of the rate of metabolism. The thyroid hormones are the regulators, though just how they do so is not fully understood. But if thyroid function is inadequate, the energy production by the body will be inadequate.

Many individuals have this problem. **Unfortunately, basic misunderstandings on thyroid function exist in the medical community** which block the help which would otherwise be available to solve many of the health problems of our nation.

The ignorance in the medical community concerning thyroid needs to be overcome. Will Rogers once said, "Ignorance ain't our problem, it's all we know that ain't true." Unfortunately all we know about hypothyroidism in the medical field "ain't" true. In fact, most of the information, particularly the thyroid blood tests being relied upon by the medical profession, is wrong. Scientists have seldom been open minded when their cherished ideas are challenged. Almost all theories that have challenged the status quo have had major hurdles to face before they were accepted. Great names in medicine such as Pasteur and Salk faced disrespect and negativity from their colleagues. I, too, have faced opposition in my approach to thyroid problems, an approach I received from Dr. Broda Barnes.

Dr. Broda Barnes rejected the accuracy of the traditional blood tests in the diagnosis of thyroid problems. Also, synthetic T4 thyroid preparations are used almost exclusively by most of the medical community, while the more effective natural desiccated thyroid products Dr. Barnes advocated, are shunned. I am writing this book in an effort to clear up some of the misconceptions fostered by the medical community. **A true understanding of the thyroid and its relationships would revolutionize medicine,** giving hope and healing to many who are facing seemingly insurmountable medical problems. A small minority of physicians recognize that another approach to thyroid problems is needed. The scientific evidence for alternative approaches to thyroid problems is growing. Thyroid hormone supplementation has an almost unbelievable impact on the health of individuals who have shown no thyroid problems on traditional thyroid blood testing. Though some of the information in this book is technical, I have tried to keep it simple enough so it can be understood by the lay person. Each chapter opens with portions from patient testimonies---only a few of the many available. Only first names have been used and these have been changed to protect the identity of these individuals. I thank each of them for permission to use their stories.

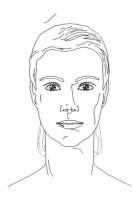

After Pauline had her last child in 1983, she began having bouts of fatigue and depression. She first sought out medical doctors and then chiropractors in an effort to gain relief from her symptoms. The only solution she was given was antidepressants, and these were only minimally effective, taking the edge off her depression but leaving the fatigue untouched. A complete blood work up, including a hypothyroid panel, was normal. She noted other symptoms: her hair was falling out, she had mood swings, suffered from insomnia, and was having problems with her normally sharp memory. Her legs were restless and she could not drive any distance without having to stop and walk around to relieve this restlessness. Her vision was deteriorating. Her singing voice changed. From a range of three octaves it narrowed down to one and one half octaves. Every year she had a physical exam with blood tests. Every year the blood tests for her thyroid hormones came back as normal. In 1990 she slowly started to gain weight and she gradually put on thirty pounds. New symptoms developed. She felt a pressure in her throat. Her heart began to race frequently. She was given a stress test which was normal except for the fact she developed an irregular heartbeat on exercise. On a physical exam, her thyroid gland had become enlarged. A thyroid scan showed adequate function of the gland but confirmed the enlargement. After more normal blood tests, the doctor she was seeing raised the possibility of thyroid cancer. Ultrasound exams followed which showed "holes" in her gland. The surgeon she consulted reassured her, telling her this was a normal goiter pattern, a normal pattern seen with an enlarged thyroid gland. He confirmed his diagnosis of goiter with a biopsy. But she suffered six weeks of terror while her diagnostic tests were going on. After another six months of repeated normal thyroid blood testing, she was placed on the synthetic thyroid hormone, Synthyoid. The only effect she noticed from this thyroid therapy was that her slow weight gain ceased. All other troubling symptoms remained. By 1996 the goiter had increased to the size of a tennis ball. She was actually falling asleep while driving. She often would have to pull over to the side of the road and walk around to try to wake up before going on. It was then she was seen in my office and was placed on two grains of Armour Thyroid on the basis of her low basal temperature and her cluster of hypothyroid symptoms. At the time her treatment was initiated, her local family physician gave her a blood test for hypothyroidism which again turned out normal. The following month when the thyroid dosage was increased to three grains, marked improvement in her health began. She could sleep through the night, and was not falling asleep while driving. She rapidly lost six pounds. Her goiter started shrinking and was down to half its previous size. Her memory improved---she was taking college courses and making straight A's. The goiter continued to shrink and after a year it was barely noticeable. All other symptoms left except her vision did not return to normal. For fifteen years her subnormal thyroid function was missed; missed due to an unjustified reliance on blood tests for hypothyroidism by the medical profession. Pauline's story is far too common.

Her story could have been different. In the 1970's, Dr. Broda Barns wrote a book on hypothyroidism titled, *Hypothyroidism: the Unsuspected Illness.* His book has pointed thousands to the pathway of thyroid replacement therapy, therapy which has restored their health. Though this book was written nearly thirty years ago, it still has an important message. Doctors are not doing any better now in diagnosing hypothyroidism than they were then. In fact the situation has become worse over the last few years as the new generation of health care providers relies even more on blood tests to diagnosis hypothyroidism. Hypothyroidism is not suspected as the underlying cause of many illnesses for which these doctors are consulted. Even when a problem with hypothyroidism is suspected, due to the clinical presentation these patients have, the blood tests which then are run usually come back normal and the suffering patient is told he or she does not have a thyroid problem. ***But most of them indeed do have a thyroid problem!*** After being told numerous times, often by different doctors that nothing is wrong, these patients come to believe what they are told---there is nothing that can be done to help them.

If they only knew that help is available, they would search until they found it. A subtitle for this book could be *Hypothyroidism: the Misunderstood Illness.* It is obviously misunderstood because doctors are not diagnosing the vast majority of patients with hypothyroidism when they rely on the blood tests to make the diagnosis. And since they are missing the majority of patients with the problem, they do not truly appreciate the vast range of symptoms that hypothyroidism causes. The second factor in the misunderstanding of hypothyroidism is the fact that most doctors in the United States use synthetic thyroid hormones to treat patients they diagnose as hypothyroid. About 75% of doctors use the synthetic brand name *Synthroid.* *Synthroid* and the other commonly used synthetic thyroids are pure thyroxine, T4 preparations, and do not have the same effects in the body as do natural desiccated thyroid products, thyroid products from animal glands which have been purified and have had the water removed. The desiccated thyroids also have T3 which is the thyroid hormone responsible for most of the metabolic activity of the body, essential to the proper functioning of each individual cell. (T7 is more active metabolically than T3 but is present is such small quantities that it is not clinically important.) Other thyroid hormones such as T2, whose functions as yet are not well understood, are present in the desiccated products.

Many of the symptoms of hypothyroidism do not clear up completely on *Synthroid* and although some patients who take the synthetic preparations do feel better, others do not. When the synthetic preparations came out in the 1960's it was assumed they would be equivalent to the natural thyroid products and they were never tested. Actually they did not receive FDA approval, for their manufacturers assumed they did not need such approval. They believed their products were not only equivalent to the natural products but were superior. In 1997 the manufacturers of those synthetic products were told by the FDA they had to seek official approval of their products due to many problems, such as losing potency before the expiration date, that were being encountered. At present only one synthetic product has submitted its application and has been approved. The others had until August of 2001 to do so. The date was originally set at August of 2000 but was extended since none of the synthetic products qualified at that time. Likely it will be extended again. Synthroid is trying to argue that it should be exempt because of its long history of usage rather than submit any new data to the FDA.

In contrast to those taking the synthetic T4, preparations, patients taking desiccated products usually gain full relief, undoubtedly due to some of the differences in these products. The reasons will be explained later. Many doctors do not appreciate the effectiveness of treating patients fully for their hypothyroid problems that is treating them with the desiccated thyroid hormones until all their symptoms are corrected. This lack of a fully effective treatment with *Synthroid* and other synthetic thyroid preparations also leads to a misunderstanding of hypothyroidism and the problems it causes.

For example, most doctors today believe that one type of hypothyroidism,(or low thyroid function), primary hypothyroidism, which is the inability of the thyroid gland to produce or release sufficient thyroid hormones, is by far the most common type of thyroid problem. It is usually the only type considered in testing for low thyroid conditions. But it is not the most common low thyroid condition. Problems which occur with thyroid metabolism within the individual cell are far more common. These fall into two categories. *The problem of the improper conversion of T4 to the much more active T3 in the cells and the problem of thyroid resistance in which the body does not respond normally to the thyroid hormone present due to problems with the thyroid binding sites.* These kinds of problems are not detected by the blood tests in current use; unfortunately, the medical profession is usually ignorant concerning them. Actually there are at least six different conditions that lead to inadequate thyroid function in the body. Every generation for the last one hundred years has had some doctors who cry out that many hypothyroid problems are being missed with tragic consequences for health. I am joining my voice to those uttering this cry.

I believe **Hypothyroidism** may be the *single most important health problem* today; certainly it is the most important problem that is not being diagnosed. Every aspect of bodily function is touched when hypothyroidism is present, and mild degrees of hypothyroidism are very common. Dr. Broda Barnes believed that in the Denver area, where he practiced, about 40% percent of the population would benefit from being on thyroid hormones. [1] In much of the developing world where iodide is not added to the salt supply, the incidence often is much greater. In some communities more than 90% percent of the people have goiters, or enlarged thyroid glands, and most of them exhibit some of the signs of hypothyroidism. A thyroid hormone is an iodide compound and lack of iodine thus can have a devastating effect on the functioning of the thyroid gland. Those living inland tend to have less iodine in their diet than those living near the ocean. Since the use of iodized salt became generalized, the goiters that run hand in hand with a deficiency of iodine are rare in the Western world; but they still do occur, perhaps indicating some individuals need more iodine than they are receiving. The breadbasket, the wheat and corn growing areas of the United States, has soils that are low in iodine content. Other mineral deficiencies aggravate the dietary iodine lack, such as a lack of selenium, magnesium and zinc The prevalence of goiter and of hypothyroidism varies from one part of the United States to another. For example, a doctor practicing in rural Idaho[2] reported that 90% of the patients he saw were hypothyroid. Hypothyroidism is important in all parts of the United States. Dr. Broda Barnes believed that the incidence of hypothyroidism was actually increasing all over the world but particularly in the Western world.

---

[1] . Broda Barnes & Lawrence Galton **Hypothyroidism, the Unsuspected Illness** Harper & Row, Publishers New York 1976

[2] Personal communication

Hypothyroidism, where there is a deficiency of the hormone or of its function, is by far the most common thyroid problem, though hyperthyroidism where the gland releases too much thyroid hormone, occurs. Cancer of the thyroid gland is also seen, but in most individuals it tends to be low grade with long term survival usual. Even if you have no problem yourself with thyroid function, some type of thyroid problem, most often hypothyroidism will affect many people you know, and will affect their relationships and their ability to work. The fact that the diagnosis of hypothyroidism is usually missed by the medical profession is without a doubt the *biggest medical tragedy* of our day.

How often is the diagnosis of hypothyroidism missed? In the Federal Registry of November 1997, the FDA [3] gives statistics on the incidence of primary hypothyroidism. As mentioned, the medical profession believes that primary hypothyroidism is by far the most common cause of hypothyroidism. Congenital hypothyroidism is found in one child for every 4,000 births and is usually caught early. Primary hypothyroidism, which is believed by the medical profession to be the most common type of hypothyroidism, is much more common in women than it is in men. In adult men the incidence is quoted 0.3%, while in women it is 1.3%. After age sixty the incidence of hypothyroidism climbs sharply and has been increasing. In women, for example, the incidence climbs to more than 7%. in some recent studies it has climbed to 9%. This means that in young adults where it is most important to prevent the sometimes insidious ill effects of hypothyroidism, *primary hypothyroidism is actually seen in less than one individual in twenty* who could be benefitting from therapy with thyroid hormones. (We are assuming with Dr. Broda Barnes that 40% of the population has hypothyroidism that should be treated.)

Many other problems follow hypothyroidism. The thyroid is part of an intricately balanced endocrine system. A malfunctioning thyroid throws the whole endocrine system out of kilter. When treating individuals for hypothyroidism, the whole endocrine system needs to be brought back into balance. Some people are very sensitive to minor changes in thyroid levels and getting them into balance is an arduous process. Fortunately the treatment for most individuals with hypothyroidism is straightforward.

Perhaps the facts recounted give a hint as to why some thyroidologists or

---

[3] Federal Registry November 1997

doctors who specialized in disorders of the thyroid gland used to say, "understand hypothyroidism, and you will understand medicine, you will understand how the human body works". This book will demonstrate why this is true.

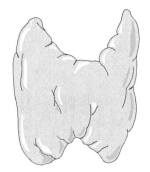

Chapter 2   The Shield Gland

Michael grew up and married the girl who lived next door. He also grew up to reach six foot seven inches in height. His dream was a career in law enforcement, and he followed his dream, eventually becoming an award winning policeman. Then his life's dream began to unravel. A drunk driver trying to run a road block at nearly eighty miles an hour knocked a parked police car into Michael. After that Michael's back and knees would

THE THYROID not allow him to continue in the police force. He had just too much pain. He still stayed in law enforcement, investigating Medicaid and Medicare fraud for the county where he lived. His childhood allergies became worse, and smog made him absolutely miserable. While still in his early fifties, he had an episode of partial paralysis and his neurologist decided he had had a light stroke. There followed a series of transient ischemic attacks, attacks in which portions of the brain did not get enough blood for short periods of time. But after numerous tests no cause for these attacks was uncovered. Michael's health continued its downward slide. He was tired and even his libido was deserting him. It was then he was diagnosed as having a hypothyroid problem along with a weak adrenal system. Though the blood tests that were run for hypothyroidism were normal, his basal temperature was very low. He was started on a combination of thyroid and adrenal support. Soon he felt like a young man again. His constant back pain and knee pain were gone, his energy returned. The transient ischemic attacks stopped. Every single symptom went away. There was an almost unbelievable improvement in Michael's health when he started taking physiologic doses of thyroid and adrenal hormones and finally reached adequate dosages of these medications.

Though the diagnosis of hypothyroidism awaited the development of modern medicine, in too many cases like Michael's, medicine today does little better in finding the problem than it did before the diagnosis of hypothyroidism even existed. Modern medicine had its roots in the science of the Reformation. Early on during the Reformation, the human body became an object of study. Anatomy was in, and the thyroid became a part of that study though the early scientists had no idea of the purpose of the gland. In 1648 it was given its name, thyroid, by Wharton, an English scientist, as a result of his own investigations in anatomy Why it received the name is no longer known. Some speculate that it was given the name because it overlies the thyroid cartilage (a part of the trachea or windpipe going into the lungs) that looks a bit like a Roman shield. Or perhaps it was due to its own shape---two oval structures joined together at the top. Thyroid is the Roman name for shield. So the thyroid gland is the "shield gland."[4]

Wharton, who gave the thyroid its name, did not realize how appropriate that name actually was. He did not realize that the hormones produced by the thyroid act as a shield warding off many chronic disease conditions that would otherwise afflict individuals. Today with a population increasing in age, there has been a corresponding increase in chronic disease---diseases such as heart disease, cancer and arthritis. The thyroid is a shield that gives protection against all these diseases. But it does far more. It protects the body against infections. And it makes life much more pleasurable.

Hypothyroidism, though it afflicted far more people was not the first thyroid disease described by modern medicine.   That honor goes to Hyperthyroidism. Hyperthyroidism, an overproduction of thyroid hormones, with its dramatic symptoms of weight loss, racing heartbeat, and weakness, was the first to be recognized historically having been first described by Parry in 1786. But its description by Grave's in 1835 made the medical profession truly aware of the condition and hyperthyroidism is still called Grave's disease. It was not until 1850 that hypothyroidism was described by Curling.   Although Hedenus removed a goiter (an enlarged thyroid gland) completely in 1800, the full development of surgery including thyroid surgery awaited the development of anesthesiology. Thyroid surgery started coming into general use in 1878, having been pioneered by Theodor Kocher, who eventually was to receive a Nobel prize for his accomplishments. Four years later in 1882, Reverdin realized he could produce hypothyroidism by removing the thyroid gland. Not until the 1890's was hypothyroidism treated with any success. At that time Murray and Howitz pioneered the use of crude thyroid extracts in its treatment. That iodine was an important part of the thyroid hormone was recognized at this time. Thyroid hormone was finally isolated by Kendall in 1914[5], and it has been an extremely important part of medicine ever since.

Nature itself hints at the thyroid's importance. Hormones are manufactured by

---

[4] Seymour I. Schwarts MD; **Principles of Surgery;**. McGraw Hill Book Company, 1967; pp. 1286-1316.

[5] Seymour I. Schwarts MD; **Principles of Surgery;** McGraw Hill Book Company, 1967.

the body and stored before they are used. Most hormone producing glands have a two to three day supply available to the body. This limited supply is not true of the hormones produced by the thyroid gland. That gland keeps a full three months' supply of hormones in reserve. Even at that, the thyroid gland does not have to store a large volume of thyroxine and liothyronine, T4 and T3, the main hormones produced by the thyroid gland. Since they are so potent, only a teaspoonful of pure thyroid hormone will keep the body's metabolism running full tilt for a year. So the thyroid gland does not have to be large. A mere twenty grams, about the size of a walnut, is its usual size. But if not enough iodine is present in the body to produce the needed T4, the thyroid gland enlarges remarkably in an effort to produce sufficient quantities of this essential hormone, resulting in a goiter.[6]

Thyroid hormones are essential for good health, though an individual can exist without a thyroid gland, at least for a time. Individuals in the late 1800s had their thyroid glands removed when large goiters were literally choking them to death. This early surgery was done before any replacement therapy was available for hypothyroidism or low thyroid function. Amazingly, these individuals survived for an average of fifteen years without any thyroid gland or no replacement therapy. The word "survived" is appropriate to describe their condition, for they could not enjoy living. They became increasingly sluggish, gained weight, spent much of their time sleeping and were emotionally unstable. Half of them developed psychotic symptoms including hallucinations.[7]

Early in the 20th century, the knowledge of thyroid increased rapidly. But the manufacture and control of thyroid hormones by the body is complex and still is not fully understood. The control process can break down at almost any point. Certain individuals are born with problems producing thyroid hormone. But these conditions are quite rare. *World wide, perhaps the most common reason that the thyroid gland does not produce sufficient thyroid hormone for the needs of the body is a lack of*

---

[6] Leslie J. Degroot; **The Thyroid and its Diseases**; Churchill Lingnston 6th Edition, 1996.

[7] Broda Barnes, & Lawrence Galton; **Hypothyroidism the Unsuspected Illness**. Harper & Row, Publishers, 1976

iodine in the diet. [8] Each molecule of thyroid hormone contains four atoms of iodine. A lack of iodine in the diet as a cause of hypothyroidism has not been a problem in the United States or Europe for a number of years. Iodized salt, salt which has iodine added, has seen to that. The soils in the bread basket of the US, the great river basins of the country, are all deficient in iodine. Non iodized salt is now available in the corner grocery store, which is a step backward, a step which may reintroduce hypothyroidism from iodine lack into this country. The importance of iodine is starting to be ignored. But since iodine compounds are used in breads and other foods as a preservative, Americans may get sufficient iodine from these sources. But if doctors see an upsurge in the incidence of goiter, and other thyroid problems as a result of the iodine lack, guaranteeing sufficient iodine intake in the diet will regain its importance. Taking extra iodine will shrink the size of a goiter, but once it is well established, the iodine may not get rid of the goiter completely. This is true both in hypothyroidism when the gland is producing too little thyroid and in hyperthyroidism, where too much thyroid hormone is being produced. Both can cause an enlarged gland. Also, some autoimmune diseases of the thyroid will increase the size of the gland, but usually not to as great a degree. In autoimmune diseases the body is turned against itself, so the body is attacking its own thyroid gland. In hyperthyroidism the shrinking of the gland caused by iodine is temporary but it is helpful if one is to have thyroid surgery as a means of treatment for hyperthyroidism. The surgery involved is a lot less bloody when the activity of the thyroid gland has been toned down.[9]

Though lack of iodine may be the commonest cause of hypothyroidism in the developing world, this is not true in the United States. The medical profession considers primary hypothyroidism to be the most common type of hypothyroidism seen here. A common underlying cause in the U.S. is the result of the treatment of other thyroid conditions, particularly hyperthyroidism. These individuals are given medications to reduce the output of a thyroid hormone by their own gland. These medications also reduce the transformation of this T 4 to the much more active T 3 hormone. This medical treatment is losing favor as a means of controlling hyperthyroidism, for it is often impossible to maintain these patients in the proper range of thyroid hormone production as measured by the blood tests. These patients suffer

---

[8] Lewis E. Braverman MD; **Werner & Ingbar's The Thyroid.** Lippincott & Ravens Publisher 7th Edition, 1996.

[9]Ibid

frequent relapses of their hyperthyroidism even when good control is achieved. For many years, surgery was the preferred method of treatment of hyperthyroidism in young women because the alternative, the use of radioactive iodine to destroy the excess activity of the thyroid gland was feared, due to possible long term side effects, particularly the fear that there might be an increase in cancer of the thyroid gland. Today radioactive iodine is the usual therapy recommended, as no evidence has been found that an increase in cancer occurs to any measurable degree.[10] It is easier than surgery and does not leave a scar. Radioactive iodine works by destroying the tissue of the thyroid gland, thus decreasing its ability to manufacture thyroid hormones.

Following either surgery or radioactive iodine therapy, most hyperthyroid patients are over corrected and become hypothyroid or low thyroid needing thyroid replacement. Although some of these individuals may be euthyroid, or have a normal thyroid function, immediately following their therapy, with the passage of time more and more of these individuals show clinical signs of hypothyroidism and show evidence of primary hypothyroidism on their blood tests. The usual explanation for the development of hypothyroidism has been that developing scar tissue chokes the remaining gland, gradually decreasing its output. The true explanation more likely is that hyperthyroidism is an autoimmune problem. In autoimmune disease, the body is fighting and gradually destroying its own tissue. Removing or destroying a portion of the thyroid gland does not change the underlying autoimmune process. As the autoimmune disease which underlies hyperthyroidism progresses, more thyroid tissue is destroyed, eventually resulting in inadequate function. It is interesting that if a careful history of hyperthyroid patients is taken, one will uncover the fact that these individuals showed signs of being hypothyroid before the onset of their hyperthyroidism. And there was an intermediate time period when they were functioning very well.

Before leaving the subject of hyperthyroidism, one more fact should be brought out. Almost all types of autoimmune disorders in the body are treated with the use of steroids. I cannot understand why steroids have not become a routine part of the treatment of all hyperthyroid patients. The medical treatment for hyperthyroidism would be much more successful if this were done. Thyroid hormones and adrenal hormones (various steroids) have functions that are intimately intertwined. The steroids

---

[10]Peter A Singer MD et. al; **Guidelines for Physicians**. American Thyroid Association, 1996.

tend to balance out some of the effects of high levels of thyroid, so steroid treatment should be even more successful than with other types of autoimmune disorders. To understand some of these relationships better, we need to briefly look at both thyroid and adrenal functions in the body.

Before talking about how thyroid functions in the body, a last cause of primary hypothyroidism needs to be discussed. The most common cause of primary hypothyroidism today is considered to be autoimmune disorders. The most common of these is HAIT or Hashimoto's thyroiditis. Most autoimmune disorders of the thyroid do not produce hyperthyroidism except perhaps for short periods of time and in a superficial way. The opposite is true; they produce hypothyroidism. As mentioned earlier, the autoimmune disorders over time gradually destroy the thyroid gland. [11] That is one of the reasons why the incidence of primary hypothyroidism is higher in individuals above sixty years of age. As they age, their glands are gradually destroyed by autoimmune disorders.

How common are the autoimmune problems of the thyroid? If one is talking about an autoimmune problem that will cause sufficient inflammation so the patient notices it, the answer is, not very common. However, auto-antibodies to thyroid hormones in the blood of patients are common. (Blood testing is the only way mild autoimmune disorder of the thyroid can be recognized. The more severe cases will have tenderness or soreness of their thyroid gland.) Twenty percent of young women develop this condition following childbirth. It is equally high in such conditions as diabetes with 10% of diabetics eventually having primary hypothyroidism show up on their blood tests. Some doctors have found that all patients with thyroid auto antibodies benefit from treatment with thyroid hormones. This is likely due to the relationship of autoimmune disease with thyroid and adrenal problems---the subject of the chapter on autoimmune disease.

How thyroid hormone works in the body is not yet fully understood. Some researchers believe that just its control of the metabolism, or heat production in the individual cells throughout the body, is enough to explain most of its effects. This idea is likely incorrect. Thyroids metabolic effects occur by regulating *how fast the body's fuel,* mainly glucose *is burned* by the individual cells of the body. It is known that thyroid hormone works in the nucleus of cells. Thyroid is involved in the transcription

---

[11]Leslie J. Degroot **The Thyroid and Its Disease.** Churchill Lingnston 1996

of information in the cell from the cell's genetic code. It is involved in the formation of all the body's proteins, and thus all its enzyme systems. Thyroid is involved in the formation of the body's neurotransmitters, the messenger molecules in the communication network of the brain. It also is active in the mitochondria, the power plants of the cell. Thyroid is involved in carbohydrate metabolism and in lipid metabolism. So thyroid is involved in all processes that take place in the body, regulating these processes through its effects on the enzymes of the body and its effects on metabolism. Disrupt the power in a factory, and all the production that takes place in that factory is affected. One can begin to see why thyroid function is so important.

The steroids also play an important role. Though steroids like prednisone and hydrocortisone are often given in clinical medicine for their role in reducing inflammation, that is not their primary function. Prednisone and hydrocortisone belong to a class of steroids called glucocorticoids. The name indicates the glucocorticoids have something to do with the metabolism of glucose and are intimately connected with many different aspects of its metabolism, including both glucose's storage and its release from body stores. For quick availability, glucose is stored as glycogen in the liver. For more sustained energy needs, protein and fat are converted into glucose or burned more directly. The glucocorticoids control, in concert with other hormones, the release of lipids from the fat stores. In a pinch the body can convert protein into glucose for burning, a process also controlled by the glucocorticoids. So thyroid hormones control the rate of burning of the fuel in the cells while the glucocorticoids regulate the availability of that fuel. Later chapters will look at these relationships in more detail.

The most important question for the individual, however, is: Does my body have enough energy to accomplish all the tasks it needs to do? Energy needs vary throughout the day. One will need far more fuel, or glucose, if one is exercising, compared to sitting and reading a book. In regulating the body's metabolism both thyroid and adrenal need to be very dynamic systems, responding to differing energy needs. If either system is off, the other will not function properly and the body will lack the energy to cope with increased demands on its resources. So the symptoms seen with either a lack of thyroid hormone or a lack of the adrenal glucocorticoids will be much alike, for both result in an inadequate production of energy. Some of the differences will be discussed later. It is evident just how important this function of controlling metabolism actually is.

Environmental Concerns:

In facing our current health challenges, the question can be asked, why are chronic diseases increasing? Certainly the increasing age of the population in Western society is a partial explanation. But age alone does not explain all the increases in chronic disease, for the rates of certain diseases seem to be increasing. Is the shield gland, thyroid, failing to protect our population from chronic diseases for some reason?

A partial answer lies in the fact that we live in a world in which we are increasingly exposed to toxins. Things that we ordinarily think of as harmless may have major deleterious consequences. For example take diet drinks with aspartame (nutrasweet) in them. When aspartame is exposed to temperatures above 86° F. it can decomposes into formaldehyde, formic acid and methanol or wood alcohol---all very toxic substances. If the factories in the body lack energy, the body will not be able to handle the toxic load and a multitude of health problems can arise, mainly in the nervous system. Also foods are frequently brought into the U. S. from foreign countries, often countries which allow the use of pesticides that are banned here. Our bodies are facing an increasingly greater challenge. They must be tuned to top efficiency if we are to remain well.

There are direct relationships with some environmental problems and thyroid. Iodine, which is a necessary part of the thyroid molecule, belongs to a family of elements called halogens. Some doctors are concerned that we are being exposed to too many other members of the halogen family in our environment and that somehow this is interfering with thyroid function. For example, two halogens are present in our water supply---chlorine and fluorine. Fluorine is known as a very toxic substance that can cause many different problems.[12] Some believe fluorine, which was added to our water supplies to try to prevent tooth decay, was added without adequate testing. Fluorine at one time was used to control hyperthyroidism. It was not necessary to ingest the fluorine---it was placed in water and the individual to be treated merely soaked in that water. So there is little question that the fluorine added to the water supply is adversely affecting thyroid function.

Chlorine has improved the safety of our water in terms of preventing infections.

---

[12]Goodman & Gillman; **The Pharmacological Basis of Therapeutics**. McGraw Hill 8th Edition, 1990.

But from time to time concerns about its use have also been raised. One of these concerns has been the possibility that chlorine might hasten the development of arteriosclerosis---hardening of the arteries. Does chlorine do so by interfering with thyroid function? Later in the book we will cite evidence that hypothyroidism is tied to the development of arteriosclerosis. No one to my knowledge has investigated this possibility. It is known that some of the compounds formed by adding chlorine to water inhibit thyroid function. Scientist are just now trying to establish safe levels for some of these substance.

Other environmental concerns on thyroid function center around mercury, which is known to be very toxic. The silver fillings that dentists put in our teeth are slightly more than 50% mercury. When combined with other metals, this mercury is still felt to be safe by most in the dental profession. But there is strong evidence that in some individuals the mercury is leaching out of the fillings and being absorbed by the body with dire consequences. Chewing accelerates its release, and a recent study in Europe noted that prolonged chewing of gum doubles the amount of mercury the body absorbs. Mercury antagonizes the actions of selenium, an important element needed for thyroid function. *Mercury also blocks the action of thyroid hormone directly, it ties up thyroid binding sites.*[13] To function, thyroid, like other molecules, has a special place within the cell that it has to attach to in order to perform its duties. Think in terms of a ball game. If the catcher does not stay behind home plate where he belongs, it spells disaster for the team. With no one to stop the ball when the pitcher throws it, all members of the opposing team will reach first base. In like manner, if mercury crowds thyroid out of its proper position, it cannot perform its functions. Thyroid function has improved greatly in some individuals when mercury is removed from their fillings, an improvement indicated by a marked increase in metabolism shown by a basal temperature that jumps as much as 1 ½ $^\circ$ F. indicating a higher rate of metabolism.

To understand other important environmental threats to the proper functioning of thyroid hormone, more information on the thyroid binding sites is helpful. Back in 1989 the medical community was surprised to learn there was a strong resemblance between thyroid binding sites which are located in the nucleus of the cells and the sites that bind certain steroid hormones. In 1997 it was discovered that estrogen binds to

---

[13]Hal A. Huggins, DDS; **It's All In Your Head,** Life Science Press, 1990.

thyroid sites quite strongly.[14]   Though men produce and utilize small amounts of estrogen, estrogen is the dominant female hormone. In women, estrogen produces the sexual characteristics of being feminine.   High levels of estrogen cut down thyroid function. This is likely the reason so many more women, about four times more, have symptomatic hypothyroidism as compared to men. But what does this have to do with the environment? It is well known that many environmental contaminants have estrogen like effects---for example many pesticides such as the outlawed DDT. (DDT, however, was safer than the pesticides now in use.) This environmental contamination has been a growing concern in the medical community and is blamed for the decreased sperm count and decreased fertility that is being seen in many men. It is probable that these contaminants are interfering with normal thyroid function by binding to thyroid binding sites. Other mechanism occur. It is known that the toxin, dioxin, interferes with brain development in the fetus by blocking thyroid function in the brain. So it is evident that the thyroid is facing numerous environmental challenges.

But for many the lack of adequate metabolism can be explained by lifestyle. Though aerobic exercise is touted for its health benefits, there is evidence that this kind of exercise tends to decrease thyroid function, likely as part of a built in feedback system which prevents the body from becoming overheated.   At body temperatures over 105 °F. brain cells begin to fry. So one can only raise body temperature about 2 ½ °F. through exercise. Likely the build up of lactic acid blocks formation of T 3, but I know of no research that has investigated this issue.

Diet is also important.   In fact all the major food groups or imbalances in them can cause hypothyroidism. Too much sugar when it causes hypoglycemia will reduce the level of T3 produced by the cells.   A diet that contains insufficient protein or protein of poor quality is known to slow metabolism.   Finally polyunsaturated fats interfere with the functioning of the mitochondria and again will slow metabolism.

Only if we give thyroid hormones to those who do not have adequate levels of the hormone will the thyroid shield hold. Only then will we start seeing a decrease in chronic disease. But to gain a better understanding of hypothyroidism, we need to explain how the body regulates thyroid hormone levels. We will also examine some

---

[14]Roderick E. M. Scott et. al. ; **Interactions of Estrogen and Thyroid Hormone Receptors.** Neurobiology & Behavior 1997; II-11 pp. 1581-1592.

.

of the symptoms produced by hypothyroidism and inadequate adrenal function.

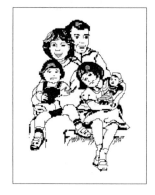

Chapter 3   Through Three Generations

Hypothyroidism can be incapacitating in the problems it causes and can inflict succeeding generations. Let Elaine tell her story.

In 1964, while engaged to be married and working as a registered nurse at Nebraska Methodist Hospital in Omaha, Nebraska, I felt that my energy did not keep up with other normal people. By evening, I was usually exhausted and felt like staying home rather than going out with my friends. After our marriage in 1965, my husband noticed that I tended to be colder than others around me. Following the birth of our first child in 1966, I began to experience chronic stuffy nose, irritability and continued fatigue. During an appointment with an internist, also a teacher at UCLA Medical School, I was diagnosed as being low thyroid---though my test was low normal, he thought I would feel better on a little thyroid. A little Synthroid did help my energy and stuffy nose for several years. Occasionally it gave me a hyper feeling and made me nervous as well. In 1970, being young and foolish, I decided I didn't want to depend on medication anymore, threw away my pills and forgot about them for the next seven years.

Each successive year after stopping the thyroid, I felt a little more tired, but it happened so slowly that I didn't get the connection. I began to develop some allergic reactions. We were living overseas at the time when I became violently allergic to a papaya---was hospitalized for severe abdominal pain and vomiting. By 1977 when we returned to the States, I was so fatigued that other family members were doing most of the work for me. Before we had a chance to actually see a doctor and get medical testing, one night I was awakened by a terrible spell of tachycardia and chest pain. The next day I had a complete cardiac work up at St. Luke's Hospital in Denver and was sent home with a monitor. All test results were negative. Later I was hospitalized for more complete testing. All the thyroid tests were negative. I became extremely weak, could barely raise my arms to comb my hair. The spells of rapid heart beat and chest pain continued. When I walked, there was heavy pressure on my chest. The least excitement, good or bad, would start my heart racing. It was hard to swallow. My neck was sore from my throat down the sternum. Almost every night I would awaken in the early morning hours, shaking all over, and with rapid heart beat and weakness that would last an hour or two. We found that benadryl, an antihistamine, seemed to blunt the reaction some, so suspected allergies were involved. When riding in the car, exhaust fumes made my chest tighten and a knot would form in my throat. When going to the store, I felt I was suffocating or going to pass out.

Since traditional medicine was not providing any answers except, "it's all in your head," we began to look for alternative routes. An osteopathic doctor diagnosed me with many food sensitivities. There was significant improvement when I limited my diet, but I was down to a handful of foods I could actually eat without getting symptoms. Besides the weakness, and rapid heart beat, I would get numbness and tingling in my extremities, extreme weakness and dizziness if I lifted my arms above my head. When I walked, I tottered because I felt my body was trembling. I had bad reactions to most medications and supplements. The osteopathic doctor started me on adrenal cortical extract shots. Within one day after my first shot, I was back to normal. I went out in the yard and pulled weeds and scrubbed the kitchen floor. In about three weeks, the shot wore off and my symptoms returned. I was given another shot and returned quickly to normal. Suddenly that year, 1978, the FDA took adrenal cortical extract off the market, not because it was dangerous, but because they claimed it was obsolete and no longer needed since the advent of cortisone. So I returned to being an invalid again.

In 1979 my husband got a hold of the book, ***Hypothyroidism the Unsuspected Illness***, by Broda Barnes. We remembered my history of hypothyroidism. My husband had me try a little synthroid and I had a violent reaction to it---thought I would die, I experienced tachycardia, almost passed out, etc.. I was afraid to try anything else, was practically an invalid and was getting tired of being incapacitated. I never gave up hope that we would find the answer somewhere, sometime. Then my husband suggested I could try a tiny bit of cortisone. No! I would never do that. I remembered all the warnings about the dangers of cortisone I had learned in nurses' training. Gradually I grew more impatient with the life of an invalid, a life of uselessness. My husband took me to see Dr. Barnes who was still practicing in Fort Collins, Colorado at the time. I knew what was coming and I dreaded it. He would put me on a little thyroid and prednisone and then I would be stuck on it the rest of my life. I rebelled against having to be dependant on a medication all my life. But I wanted to be normal and have a quality life even more. When he finished the history and physical, he prescribed the small dose of 1 gr. of Armour Thyroid and 5 mg. of prednisone.

I was feeling sorry for myself and said, "Will I have to be on this the rest of my life?"

He said, "You want to eat, don't you? "

Well, that made sense to me. Within a few days, I was eating meat which had bothered my digestion for almost a year. I gradually added more foods and gradually gained strength. The horrible spells of tachycardia disappeared, the numbness and tingling in the arms and legs went away. I no longer had dizziness or weakness when I reached up with my arms. I could do normal housework. Formerly a trip in the car or to the shopping center gave me headaches, stomachaches, generalized aching and fatigue. Now those symptoms gradually improved. There were still some foods and situations I had to avoid, but gradually my life became more normal.

It took about five years to get back to nearly full health. Even after that I improved. At first I was very sensitive to the thyroid --every time I tried to increase the dose, I would get more allergies. Gradually I found my ideal dosage was 10 mg. prednisone and 3 grs. of thyroid. On less prednisone, I became weak and short of breath when walking. On less than 2 grs. thyroid, I would space out when driving and loose my concentration. I now work an eight-hour day, and I am involved in many other activities away from work and home. I have not had any major surgeries as most women my age have had. My bone scan is still in the normal range. A few years ago I started natural progesterone and got rid of all my PMS and have felt much calmer overall. I usually can keep going to 11:00 PM at night before going to bed and awaken by 6:00 or 7:00 AM. At 5 mg of prednisone I could not take vitamin and mineral supplements; at 10 mg. I can take most supplements and medications if needed without any reactions.

In the Physicians Desk Reference, the PDR , it says when you start a patient on thyroid, check the adrenal gland to make sure there is no insufficiency. If there is adrenal insufficiency (and be aware there are different degrees of this), and you do not support the adrenal while adding the thyroid you can actually kill the patient by throwing them into adrenal crisis. Such a severe reaction is rare, most people just feel worse having symptoms like weakness, nervousness, feeling keyed up, low blood pressure, nausea, food or chemical sensitivities, rapid heart beat, etc. I have found I cannot take my thyroid without adrenal support. So doctors have told me, I have what is called **secondary** hypothyroidism, which is a diagnosis many doctors are missing today. When the TSH is low, the doctor usually says the patient has too much thyroid, because the pituitary is suppressed by the excess thyroid so this is producing the low TSH levels. However, in secondary hypothyroidism, the pituitary can't produce enough TSH to allow the thyroid to put out sufficient thyroid hormone. With thyroid and prednisone I can lead a nearly normal life; without this therapy I would be a cripple.

Elaine's mother, Brenda, was in her sixties when Elaine was diagnosed by Dr. Barnes as hypothyroid. As a result of learning her daughter was hypothyroid, she began looking at some of her own health problems. She often woke up tired and remained tired throughout the day. To have energy to do her evening chores, she would need to nap during the day. She blamed this tiredness on the fact that she was getting older. But she was also cold, colder than those around her. She was plagued by dry, itchy skin which would at times break out into a severe eczema that covered her whole body. In fact, the rash had become so severe on two separate occasions that she had been hospitalized to bring the rash under control. Her fingernails were splitting and her hair was dry, brittle and tended to fall out. She noted problems concentrating and often was tense and irritable. Her ankles tended to swell. At times she felt dizzy and had a number of fainting spells.

But her biggest problem was her breathing. She had developed asthma about ten years earlier and her asthma had been getting worse. She had four recent hospitalizations for a combination of pneumonia and asthma. Some of these episodes had been life threatening.

She was diagnosed as low thyroid and started on both adrenal support and Armour Thyroid, a natural desiccated thyroid preparation. As her asthma attacks gradually subsided, she was able to give up the respiratory therapy she had needed on a regular basis. Nearly twenty years have gone by and she has not had to be hospitalized again. Though she still has problems with eczema from time to time, her skin improved considerably when her thyroid dosage was increased to 3 grs. per day. Other than having problems with her feet stemming from complications from bunion surgery, she is in good health. In fact she is healthier now at eighty nine years of age than she was twenty years ago.

Elaine's daughter, Joy, inherited her mother's thyroid problem. The first indication of problems to come was when as a six-year-old she was living with her parents in the Orient and came down with a primary case of tuberculosis. She had to be treated for six months with isoniazide, INH, the most widely used medication for

TB. By age ten when her mother was diagnosed with *secondary hypothyroidism*, it was obvious that Joy too was going to have problems. She was developing allergies, but of more significance she was having muscle aches and pains. She had frequent stomachaches after eating. But her headaches truly plagued her. These were so severe she would scream with the pain they were causing. She showed other signs of hypothyroidism. She was tired most of the time and it would take her a whole day to finish a simple job like dust the house. She was started on natural desiccated thyroid and adrenal support. Her headaches disappeared and she became her usual happy, cheerful self. Her energy level was restored to normal. Blood tests taken since then have shown a low TSH, often in the range seen in hyperthyroidism but with a normal T4 level, a pattern consistent with secondary hypothyroidism. Blood tests taken when she was a teenager showed nonspecific autoimmune antibodies. Yet any significant autoimmune problem remains quiescent. She remains in good health while taking thyroid and prednisone. She was inconsistent in taking her medications through her college years and symptoms started returning until she became more faithful in taking them. She is now in her late twenties with two children of her own. Her own children are starting to show signs that they too may benefit from thyroid therapy before long.

This story not only illustrates many of the symptoms that can be seen in hypothyroidism, it also shows that thyroid problems often run in families. An interesting sidelight to this is the fact that it is common for both husband and wife to have a problem with hypothyroidism. The reason for this seems to be that people tend to marry others who have the same energy level. A hypothyroid individual cannot keep up with someone with normal thyroid function, someone who is bursting with energy. And the offspring of such a union (two hypothyroid individuals) will usually be hypothyroid as well.

Hypothyroidism can wear many different guises. Since hypothyroidism affects every part of the body, well over one hundred symptoms have been associated with it. Thyroid affects the production of the enzyme systems underlying the functioning of the body, so if there is an inherited or acquired weakness in any system, this weakness shows up, creating symptoms.[15] One sees a number of different clinical pictures associated with hypothyroidism for different symptoms are often present and different symptoms dominate in different individuals. Often hypothyroidism causes symptoms

---

[15]Broda O. Barnes & Lawrence Galton **Hypothyroidism the Unsuspected Illness**. Thomas Crowell Company, New York 1976

that are opposite from one another---a hypothyroid patient can be either short or tall, fat or skinny, lethargic or hyperactive. Sometimes hypothyroidism is not suspected since it causes symptoms that are not associated with the condition in the thinking of most medical personnel. Since thyroid and adrenal functions are intertwined, the symptoms that are caused by adrenal weakness are similar to those caused by hypothyroidism. It is important to know if adrenal weakness exists for, if it does, treating with thyroid alone will make a patient worse. **So a cardinal rule of treating thyroid patients is if the treatment with thyroid seems to make the patient worse in any way, add adrenal support**. It is helpful to know what symptoms tend to differentiate an individual who just has hypothyroidism from the individual who also has a significant weakness of his adrenal gland. In this chapter we will give some common clinical presentations of hypothyroidism. Then the clinical symptoms will be divided into groups to indicate which ones may point to an adrenal weakness.

Both adrenal problems and thyroid problems may share the same underlying cause. Prolonged stress puts pressure on the adrenal glands. But stress from either accident or illness is often the factor that pushes an individual into symptomatic hypothyroidism. Just the birth of a child is sufficiently stressful to do this. After the birth of her child, a mother often feels depressed. She is not able to lose the weight she gained through pregnancy. She feels tired, but blames the tiredness on having to get up at night to feed her baby. She may be sluggish mentally, may notice her skin is dry and her hair has lost its luster and seems to be falling out. These symptoms frequently get blamed on the normal aftermath of pregnancy and on the fact she is staying up at night to care for her child. The weight of the baby, particularly of the first born child may be a tip off to hypothyroidism, as a birth-weight of more than eight pounds is strongly correlated with hypothyroidism in the mother.

Another time of high stress is the teenage years. The child who was a model citizen becomes unruly and moody. She (problems are more common in girls) may be hyperactive and may actually lose weight. But teenage girls think skinny is beautiful so the fact that there is a weight problem is usually missed. All her problems may start after major dental work. She doesn't feel well after the visit to the dentist, but she has no specific complaints. As a typical teenager she may not share her feelings. Her grades drop in school. Though she remains active, if she does not get enough sleep, her behavior becomes worse and she may lose her temper with slight provocation. She has a hard time staying warm and starts wearing socks to bed at night and is always asking for the thermostat to be turned up.

And these repeated infections certainly stress the body. Severe eczema is also a tip off. Most hypothyroid individuals, whether adult or child, will be cold and tired. Many will have problems with their skin and hair. Most will also have problems with concentration or some other mental abnormality.

Though not absolute, the list on the following page will help diagnose hypothyroidism and also give an indication whether adrenal function has been impaired as well.

LOW THYROID	LOW THYROID & ADRENAL	LOW ADRENAL
Overweight	Normal Weight	Underweight
Slow Pulse	Normal Pulse	Fast Pulse
Short or Tall	Variable	Short
BP above 100 systolic	Variable low or high	BP below 100 systolic
Paresthesias (changed sensations)	Basal Temperature below 97.8° F. (Also low thyroid or adrenal)	
Chronic fatigue Starting in the afternoon	Chronic fatigue	Chronic fatigue Starting on arising
No energy	Immune system suppressed	No Stamina
Constipation	Dyspepsia, Indigestion, Hypoglycemia	Diarrhea
Dry Skin	Skin rashes	Bronze coloration
Dry Eyes	Allergies	Chemical sensitivities
Split fingernails	Asthma	Food sensitivities
Elevated cholesterol	Depression, Mood swings	Fibromyalgia
Dry brittle hair, hair falls out	Panic attacks	
Fibroid tumors	Mental illness	Autoimmune disease
Spontaneous abortion	Infertility	Need nine hour or more sleep
Toxemia	Poor memory, Concentration	
Tinnitus, Deafness	Difficulty pronouncing words	Fainting
Hoarse, Lump in Throat	Nervousness	
Difficulty swallowing	Short of breath	Chronic Fatigue Syndrome
Clumsy, Poor coordination	Cold extremities	Weakness
Abnormal sweating	Menstrual irregularities	
Anemia	Arthritis, Fibromyalgia	Thyroid increases symptoms

When an individual comes into the office complaining of symptoms consistent with hypothyroidism, the form seen below can be used to record their symptoms. All the problems noted on the form on the following page are common in hypothyroidism and if a number of them are present one should suspect that hypothyroidism is present. If the basal temperature is also low, the diagnosis is confirmed. The items listed as general are not as significant as the others and are the least important questions on this form. Those who have a number of the problems listed on the other parts of the form usually have a problem with hypothyroidism. Depression, coldness, and energy problems are of particular importance since these problems tend to make life miserable for individuals.

SAMPLE HYPOTHYROID
QUESTIONNAIRE

Patient's Name_____   Date_____

Hypothyroidism---check list:

Number your answers when appropriate as follows:
0 = almost never 1= occasional 2= often 3= almost always

1. Metabolism:

What is your basal temperature? _____Do your hands feel cold at times? _____Feet?
_____ Do you feel cooler than others around you? _____ Do your hands or feet tend
to swell? _____ Are you overweight? How much?_____ Are you underweight? How
much?_____ Do you have a high cholesterol level ? _____   Do you suffer from
constipation?____ Diarrhea_____ Do you have symptoms of low blood sugar?_____
Any frontal headaches?_____

2. Energy level:

Do you wake up tired? _____ Do you feel tired all the time? _____ Do you get more
tired than you used to?_____ Do you feel listless by afternoon? _____ After you eat?
_____ Do you have sufficient energy to do your chores efficiently in the evening? _____
Do you nap? ____ How many hours of sleep do you need to feel your best?_____ Do
you have sufficient energy to engage in an exercise program? _____ Do you have
problems going to sleep? _____ Waking up during the night?

3. Skin, Hair & Nails:

Do you have dry skin? _____ Do you have a problem with rashes? _____ Did you
as a child?_____ Do you have a problem with acne? _____ Did you as a teenage?
_____ Are your finger nails slow growing? Yes___No____ Brittle? _____ Split?
_____ Is your hair dry? ____ Brittle? _____ Does it tend to fall out? _____ More
coarse?_____

4. Women Only:

Are your periods regular? _____ Are they heavy or prolonged? _____ Any clots or cramping? _____ Do you get mood swings or any other PMS symptoms? _____ Any associated headaches? _____ Any problems getting pregnant?____ Miscarriages?_____

5. Mental :

Do you have problems with concentration? _____ With memory ? _____ With initiative? _____ With anxiety? _____ With tension? _____ With irritability? _____ With depression? _____ Do you have difficulty pronouncing words?_____

6. General:

Is there a history of thyroid disease in your family?_____ Heart disease?_____ Have you been told you have angina? (Pain that comes from the heart) _____ Have you had episodes of rapid or irregular heart beats?____ Have you had an abnormal electrocardiogram?_____How does your blood pressure run? High?_____ Low?_____ Your pulse? Fast?____ Slow?_____ Any problem with anemia?_____ With your hearing?_____ Ringing in your ears?_____ Any dizzy spells?_____ Do you have protruding eyes?____ Swelling around your eyes or eyelids?_____ Are your eyes often bloodshot?_____ Is your vision blurred?_____ Do you have dyspepsia or indigestion?____ Do you feel nauseated frequently? _____ Have you had problems with your gall bladder? _____ Do you have excess saliva?_____ Do you feel you need to clear your throat?____ Has your voice become more hoarse?_____ Any difficulty swallowing?_____Any pain or swelling around your thyroid gland?____Do you feel like you have a hard time breathing?_____ Do you have numbness or tingling of any part of your body?_____ Do your ankles swell or do you notice an other evidence of body fluid retention?____ Any abnormal sweating?____

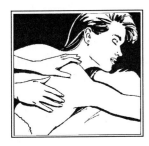

Chapter 4   The Physical Exam

It was obvious Joe had a problem. He was overweight. He moved in slow motion. Not only did he move slowly, he spoke and thought slowly as well. Just looking at him should have been enough to alert doctors to his problem, his hypothyroidism. But numerous tests, including thyroid tests, had come back normal, so his symptoms and his appearance were disregarded. This went on for a dozen years. His symptoms became worse until just going to work became an almost impossible task. Joe had a low basal temperature to go along with his other symptoms. He was diagnosed as low thyroid and placed on thyroid replacement therapy. His thyroid dosage was gradually increased until he was on five grains of thyroid---an indication that his absorption of the thyroid was off or that auto-antibodies were destroying part of the thyroid before it could be used by the body. His testosterone levels were low as well, the aftermath of a bout with mumps as a young man. Testosterone was added to his regimen. His symptoms gradually improved. Though he continued to have some unrelated health problems, he became a functional human being again, able to earn a good living.

Joe's appearance was a tipoff to his thyroid problem. Just as there are many symptoms that point to hypothyroidism, there are clues that can be picked up on a physical exam, clues that point to the diagnosis as well. Some, like eczema, overweight, and sluggish movements, can be spotted some distance away. Most physical signs are merely suggestive and one needs to have a cluster, a group of signs and symptoms in order to make a diagnosis for any condition in the practice of medicine. This is certainly true of hypothyroidism.

Systematic observations need to be made in evaluating an individual with suspected hypothyroidism. In the physical exam one of the first observations is height. Hypothyroidism is associated with men more than six feet in height or less than five feet four inches---those who are more than four inches above or four inches below average range of height. Women are about four inches shorter than men so the normal range for them would be five feet to five feet eight inches. Next, the way the individual moves needs to be observed. Clumsiness and slowness of movement tend to run with low thyroid conditions. Another clue that can be seen at a distance is hair color---redheads are frequently low thyroid. Even a lot of reddish highlights in the hair may be suggestive. Premature graying of hair is also associated with a low thyroid condition, gray hair often starting before age thirty. Coarse, dry, lifeless hair is also a mark of hypothyroidism as is thinning hair. Male pattern baldness, however, has nothing to do with hypothyroidism. Thinning or loss of the outer third of the eyebrows is a common manifestation of hypothyroidism.

The way the individual talks, slowness of speech, a tendency to stumble over words can provide clues to hypothyroidism as well. If hypothyroidism is marked, the voice may be hoarse. Then a coarsening of features occurs at times resulting in a dullness of expression. This is often coupled with slight puffiness around the eyes from fluid retention. The eyes may be unusually dry and therefore may be irritated, or blood shot. Since allergies are common, dark circles may be present around the eyes from congested blood vessels.

Other things that can be seen at a glance are the appearance of rashes, particularly acne. Either a current outbreak of acne or old scarring can tip one off to the possibility of hypothyroidism. Vitiligo, a skin condition where patches of skin have lost their pigmentation, is also suggestive. Skin color can be a tip off as well. Since circulation is decreased to the skin in hypothyroidism, the skin tends to be pale. Often the liver is unable to convert beta carotene into active Vitamin A and the skin takes on a yellowish hue as a result. If adrenal insufficiency is pronounced, the skin can have an artificial bronzed appearance.

Shaking the patient's hand can be informative. That will demonstrate whether or not his extremities are cool. If the hands are clammy, this may indicate abnormal sweating. Since arthritis is more common in hypothyroidism, any deformity of joints should be noted. One can also observe the finger nails: are they short, split or in other ways show poor growth.

The vital signs need to be checked. Weight is important---hypothyroid patients tend to be overweight due to decreased metabolism, though they can be underweight as well due to poor absorption of nutrients when they eat. Temperature is extremely important. Though there are a few medications that can lower body temperature, they likely do so by interfering with thyroid or adrenal function. Both low thyroid and low adrenal states will cause a low temperature by lowering metabolism. It does not matter which is the primary problem, for low thyroid function often will result in low adrenal output, and inadequate amounts of the glucocorticoids in turn will slow thyroid function. So both conditions are often present with a low basal temperature. An oral daytime temperature should range from 98.6° to close to 100° F.. On initiation of therapy we prefer having a basal temperature. It is an important guideline in that if individuals are placed on an excessive dose of thyroid hormone, the temperature should become elevated within two weeks time. However, if the thyroid feedback mechanisms are working properly it is impossible to make an individual hyperthyroid until they are given more thyroid than the gland produces---about 4 ½ grs. for a small individual and about 5 grs. for the usual adult. Their basal temperature should rise up over 98.2° F if they are truly hyperthyroid, and thus have too much thyroid hormone.[16] The pulse is important as well; a slow pulse is typical of a pure low thyroid condition. With low adrenal function, the pulse speeds up and a rapid pulse may indicate inadequate adrenal support. The blood pressure is also an important guide line. A blood pressure with a systolic below one hundred indicates inadequate adrenal support. It is interesting to note that blood pressure often falls with illness as inadequate adrenal reserve shows up when one is ill. Even an ordinary illness often increases the need for adrenal hormones five fold.

The relationship of hypothyroidism to other health problems often provides clues to the presence of hypothyroidism in the physical exam. Hypothyroidism is an underlying cause of deafness, thus hearing problems can indicate a thyroid problem. So hearing tests can be important. Signs of chronic infections are important. Scarring of the eardrum can indicate frequent ear infections in the past. Serous otitis, which is a collection of fluid behind the ear drum, is important from the standpoint of diagnosing either a weakened immune system or the presence of allergies. Since chronic sinus infections are extremely common in those who are hypothyroid, one should observe the patient for post nasal drainage and changes in the mucous membranes of the nose, both indications of sinus infections. Though the tongue may be enlarged in hypothyroidism, this is difficult to observe unless the hypothyroidism is quite severe.

Although enlarged nodes in the neck can indicate the presence of low grade infections, particularly in the sinuses, the examination of the thyroid gland itself is the important part of the neck exam. Tenderness of the thyroid gland, which lies just below the voice box, or the larynx indicates thyroiditis, an autoimmune problem with the thyroid. Occasionally the tenderness is the result of an acute viral infection. Thyroiditis is often missed on physical exams. Enlargement of the gland or nodules

---

[16] Broda O. Barnes & Lawrence Galton; **Hypothyroidism the Unsuspected Illness**, Thomas Crowell Company, New York, 1976.

in the thyroid gland can indicate either hypothyroidism or hyperthyroidism. A single nodule can indicate cancer of the thyroid gland. Most cancers of the thyroid are slow growing and not very aggressive. Any rapidly growing nodule should be checked immediately to make sure it is not cancerous. The usual cause of such enlargement is simply bleeding into a small thyroid cyst which then suddenly enlarges and becomes a nodule one can feel, a nodule which often is tender.

The texture of the skin needs to be checked, for the skin is dry and thickened in hypothyroidism. The skin of the fingers may actually crack and bleed. At times patches of dry, rough skin will be observed elsewhere on the body, particularly during the winter. If hypothyroidism is mild, just the skin over the elbows and knees may be involved, so this is the best place to check for rough, dry skin.

There are changes in pulmonary function in hypothyroidism, but they are subtle enough that they will not be picked up on a physical exam. Of course asthma, if present, will indicate an allergy which often speaks of adrenal weakness. Both hypothyroidism and low adrenal function can produce arrhythmia of the heart. Skipped beats are common. At times atrial fibrillation---a condition in which the pacemaker of the heart is firing rapidly and wildly, resulting in an irregular heart beat---can be seen. This condition is common in hyperthyroidism and has traditionally been associated with it rather than hypothyroidism. Heart size is also affected, with the size being increased in hypothyroidism but decreased in adrenal insufficiency. Usually the size cannot be determined accurately enough to be helpful as a physical clue. Poor circulation with associated poor pulses in the extremities are tied to arteriosclerosis and to possible underlying hypothyroidism.

With the gastrointestinal problems that are frequent in hypothyroidism, vague abdominal tenderness may be found on a physical exam. The classic abdominal signs of gall bladder disease would indicate a possible thyroid problem, since the poor cholesterol metabolism associated with hypothyroidism often results in gall bladder problems. But such findings are not common enough to be helpful. The congestion of the liver often seen in hypothyroidism is not evident on a physical exam of the abdomen. Bowel sounds, the noises made by normal functioning of the intestines, tend to be sluggish in hypothyroidism and increased in hyperthyroidism, but the normal range of these sounds is so broad that these sounds are not helpful from a clinical standpoint.

In the genitourinary systems, any signs of infection may indicate that the immune function of the body is decreased. There is a high correlation between an inadequate thyroid function and poor immune function. But examination of the genitourinary system is not considered helpful in diagnosing thyroid conditions.

The neurologic exam can be significant, however. Carpal tunnel syndrome, a numbness of the fingers caused by pressure on the median nerve as it passes into the hand, is often associated with hypothyroidism. Abnormal skin sensations, or paresthesias, are again often associated with hypothyroidism. The ankle reflexes, the ankle jerks have long been used as an indicator of hypothyroidism. The relaxation phase is slowed after the tendon is tapped and shortens in response. Having the patient kneel on a chair makes it easier to observe the ankle reflexes accurately.

Finally hypothyroidism causes a puffiness of the ankles that can best be observed around the Achilles tendon. The physical features in this area will be obscured in hypothyroid patients. These landmarks will reappear with correction of the hypothyroid condition.

Though the physical signs are not used by themselves in a diagnosis of hypothyroidism, they can add valuable clues that the condition does indeed exist. All hypothyroid patients should exhibit some of the signs.

Below is a form that can be used to record the common findings seen in a hypothyroid patient on physical exam.

INITIAL FORM FOR THYROID DISEASE

Date_____

Vital Signs:

Height_____ Weight_____Temperature_____ Pulse_____Blood Pressure_____

General Appearance: Alert___ Dull____Drowsy____Clumsy____Abnormal Gait_____

Hair: Red_____Red High Lights_____ Gray_____ Thin_____ Coarse_____Balding_____

Skin: Pale_____Reddish_____Yellowish hue_____Bronzed_____Coarse_____Thin_____

Acne_____ Acne scars_____ Rash_____ Dry_____Pigment Loss_____

Ears: Serous Otitis____Scarring____Infected____

Eyes: Dry____Tearing____Bloodshot_____Periorbital Edema_____Nystagmus_____

Nose: Dark Circles_____Congested_____

Oral: Silver fillings____PND____Injection____Tongue Enlarged____Canker Sores____

Neck: Nodes____

Thyroid: Normal_____Enlarged____ Tender_____ Nodules_____

Chest: Wheezing_____Rales_____ Normal Breath Sounds_____

Heart: Regular Rhythm_____ Murmurs_____ Enlarged_____

Abdomen: Tender_____ Bowel Sounds: Hypo____Hyper____Normal____

Extremities: Cool_____Hot_____ Clammy_____

Circulation: Mildly Decreased_____Marked Decrease_____Edema_____

Reflexes: Ankle: Increased_____Normal_____Decreased_____Slow_____

Neurologic: Paresthesias_____Nerve entrapment_____

Other:_____

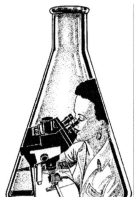

Chapter 5   Thyroid Metabolism

Sandra didn't realize she had a hypothyroid problem. "Oh, yes, I'm tired", she would say. "I'm not able to get my chores done though still young. But, after all, I do have a family to look after and they keep me on the go most of the time." Then a neighbor was treated for hypothyroidism. Seeing the difference it made in the neighbor's life made Sandra wonder if she too might have a thyroid problem. "I'll go to the same doctor as my neighbor and see." She did. She was checked out, and found to have a low basal temperature to go with her other symptoms. The thyroid supplementation she was started on soon made her realize that the tiredness she had lived with was not natural. Soon she was saying, "I'm not only keeping up with my family, but am able to reach outside my home to minister to the needs of others as well."

Like Sandra, patients on thyroid soon find that their metabolism, their body's ability to work is the key to their own ability to work, and to reach many of their goals as well. The metabolism of thyroid is complex and designed with a number of checks and balances in it. I will concentrate on areas that have important clinical implications. The actual manufacture of thyroid hormone by the thyroid gland is rarely a source of clinical problems, so the chemical details of this process will be skipped.

Thyroid is an iodine compound. Lack of iodine will produce goiter---a general enlargement of the thyroid gland either containing homogenous tissue or nodules which often can be felt on physical examination of the gland. A goiter with a single nodule can be cancerous, though a gland with multiple nodules rarely is. If a nodule is felt, the paired thyroid glands need to be examined carefully to see if other nodules are present. In some parts of the third world, particularly those lacking a seacoast, lack of iodine is the most common recognized cause of hypothyroidism. Since most salt purchased in grocery stores in the USA has iodine added, marked iodine deficiency is no longer common in the West. However, table salt is now available which has no iodine. In addition, the advice to cut salt intake given to many individuals with high blood pressure or heart disease, may play a role in the increased hypothyroidism seen in the elderly, though it is more likely due to an overall decline in hormone activity in the aging individual. While too little iodine stimulates the thyroid gland, an oversupply tends to shut the thyroid down, at least on a temporary basis. For this reason, iodine is often given to hyperthyroid patients in order to decrease the activity of the gland, reduce its blood supply and shrink the size of the gland before thyroid surgery is undertaken.

Once thyroid hormone is manufactured by the thyroid gland, the hormone released into the bloodstream is controlled by a feedback mechanism involving the hypothalamus and the pituitary gland. The medical profession

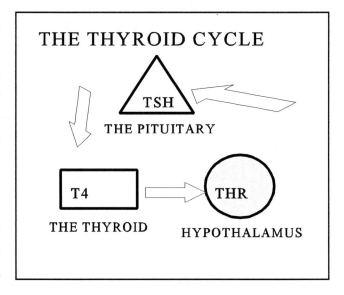

Figure 1   Feed Back Cycle

has placed its focus on thisfeed back cycle. (*Figure 1*) The blood tests we have for measuring thyroid hormone also look at elements of this feed back cycle. As a consequence, in the medical literature thyroid problems have been defined in terms of this cycle.[17] Perhaps the easiest way to visualize the thyroid cycle is in terms of the furnace in one's home. Since thyroid hormone is involved in metabolism or the heat production of the body, the analogy is apt. One can have problems with production and release of thyroid hormone from the thyroid gland. These problems are referred to as primary hypothyroidism. This is like having problems with the propane tank, the storage tank for the gas for the furnace. One can have problems relating to the function of the pituitary. The pituitary is like the **control center** which regulates the amount of gas being released from the propane tank. A malfunctioning pituitary will cause **secondary hypothyroidism,** since inadequate amounts of TSH, thyroid stimulating hormone are produced. A variety of other abnormalities can also occur. (see Table 2) TSH signals the thyroid gland to release its thyroid hormones, its T4 and T3. It is called secondary because there is nothing wrong with the thyroid gland. In our analogy it is as if there is enough gas in the propane tank, but the control system is fouled up so that not enough gas is released from the tank. Severe malfunction of the pituitary is uncommon; however, subtle malfunction is common. This subtle hypothyroidism is usually not discovered because tests are not run to analyze the functioning of the anterior pituitary gland, which can be done by examining its response

---

[17] L. Ross McDougall; **Thyroid Disease in Clinical Practice**. Oxford University Press, New York 1992.

to THR, the thyrotropic hormone from the hypothalamus.

Malfunction of the hypothalamus results in **tertiary hypothyroidism**. This is like having the thermostat malfunction in the heating system of the house. The hypothalamus releases THR or thyrotrophic releasing hormone. It in turn controls the

CONDITION	T4	TSH	FUNCTION
EUTHYROID	NORMAL	VARIABLE	
PRIMARY HYPOTHYROIDISM	LOW	HIGH, NORMAL	NOT ENOUGH "GAS" PRODUCED
SECONDARY HYPOTHYROIDISM	LOW	LOW, NORMAL	CONTROL CENTER OFF
TERTIARY HYPOTHYROIDISM	LOW	LOW, NORMAL	THERMOSTAT OFF
AUTO IMMUNE	VARIABLE	VARIABLE	"WATER" IN THE "GAS" LINE
CONVERSION PROBLEM T4 TO T3	VARIABLE	VARIABLE	CONTROL OF "FURNACE" OFF
BINDING SITE PROBLEM	VARIABLE	VARIABLE	"GAS" DOES NOT ALL BURN
PRIMARY HYPERTHYROIDISM	HIGH	LOW	TOO MUCH "GAS"
SECONDARY HYPERTHYROIDISM	HIGH	HIGH, NORMAL	CONTROL CENTER SET TOO HIGH

THYROID HORMONE MALFUNCTION   Table 2

release of TSH from the anterior pituitary. Tertiary hypothyroidism is felt to be rare and likely is. When found it is usually seen in children.

One other hypothyroid problem can be picked up by the blood tests and that is the presence of **auto-antibodies to thyroid**.[18] This is a bit like having water in the gas lines, something present that can quench the furnace so that it does not burn as well. These antibodies are targeted against thyroid or thyroid tissue Since thyroid hormones can be destroyed, the amount of active thyroid hormone available to be used by the body often is decreased, thus resulting in a hypothyroid condition.[19]. Though most patients with auto-antibodies to thyroid have improvement in a number of underlying hypothyroid symptoms when placed on thyroid, the presence of auto-antibodies is more likely a marker for a hypothyroid condition rather than the real cause. Individuals with autoimmune disease have subtle abnormalities in adrenal hormone production, abnormalities which run hand in hand with hypothyroidism.

The feedback mechanism involving thyroid was the first feedback cycle to be discovered in the body. A similar feedback cycle also controls the output of adrenal hormones, so the thyroid cycle serves as a model for hormonal control in the body. Though the thyroid gland is a manufacturing unit, it is also a storage unit with about a three-month supply of thyroid ready to be released to the body. The major output of the thyroid gland is thyroxin or T4 accounting for 95% of the circulating thyroid measured in the serum. T3 makes up the majority of the remaining portion of thyroid hormone in the blood serum. Small amounts of other thyroid hormones such as RT3 and T2 are seen as well. [20]

The hypothalamus, as a monitoring station, monitors the levels of T4 brought to it. T3 also seems to be involved in the monitoring process, but to a lesser degree. The body also notes other factors such as body temperature, taking them into consideration as well in its regulatory process. However, the T4 blood level is the most important factor considered by the hypothalamic monitoring station. In response to these factors, the hypothalamus puts out differing amounts of THR (thyrotrophic releasing hormone) to indirectly lower or raise the T4 levels in the blood. It does so by its action on the anterior pituitary. THR also functions as a neurotransmitter, a transmitter of chemical signals in the brain. In the thyroid feedback cycle, however, THR signals the anterior pituitary to produce more TSH, thyroid stimulating hormone. (Another name for TSH

---

[18] Leslie J Degroot; **The Thyroid and Its Diseases**. McGraw Hill, 1996.

[19] Karlsson F. A.; **Hypothyroidism Due to Thyroid Hormone Binding Antibodies**. N.Eng J Med, 1995; 296 pp. 1196-1198.

[20] Leslie J. Degroot; **The Thyroid and Its Diseases.** Churchill Lingnston, 1996.

is thyrotrophic hormone, thus the hypothalamus is monitoring the release of thyrotrophic hormone) The lower the T4 in the blood, the greater the amount of THR is produced. A normal pituitary will more than triple its production of TSH, usually to 30 MCIU, in response to a bolus, a quick injection, of THR. The upper limits of normal for unstimulated TSH production is 4.5 MCIU. [21]

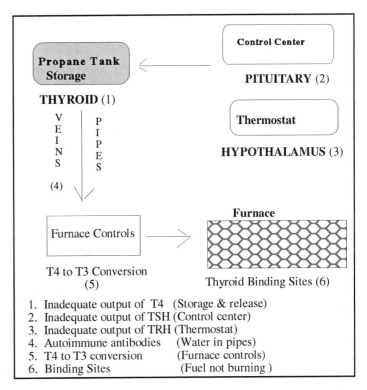

1. Inadequate output of T4   (Storage & release)
2. Inadequate output of TSH (Control center)
3. Inadequate output of TRH (Thermostat)
4. Autoimmune antibodies   (Water in pipes)
5. T4 to T3 conversion   (Furnace controls)
6. Binding Sites   (Fuel not burning)

Figure 2 Types of Hypothyroid Problems

TSH released by the anterior pituitary then signals the thyroid gland to release more thyroid hormone. Thus the blood levels of T4 are tightly controlled and cycle between fixed limits. Most endocrine glands such as the anterior pituitary put their hormones out in spurts, so the actual blood level depends upon when the last spurt occurred. Circadian rhythms, or body rhythms dependent on the time of day, are involved in hormone control. This is true for the output of TSH, so thyroid output also has a daily rhythm. Interestingly, TSH levels tend to be higher at night. Perhaps this is due to the fact that the liver does most of its repair chores at night, and the liver utilizes more thyroid hormone, particularly T3, needing a higher metabolism than any other organ in the body. Medical personnel looking at this thyroid feedback cycle have assumed that the output of the thyroid gland remains relatively constant through its twenty four-hour cycle each day. Testing of T4 levels in the blood by early researchers indicated this assumption is not true---these researchers were getting a different T4 level almost every time they checked, and some ran levels six times a day or more. So though blood levels of T4 are held within certain limits, the output of thyroid fluctuates significantly throughout

---

[21] Leslie J. Degroot; **The Thyroid and Its Diseases.** Churchill Lingnston, 1996.

the day.[22] This is just what is to be expected if the body has to adjust to the differing metabolic challenges throughout the day.   Digestion, exercise and stress all demand differing energy outputs and thus differing amounts of thyroid hormone. Subtle s e c o n d a r y hypothyroidism, subtle problems with this **feed back** and **control system** particularly with the anterior pituitary, may

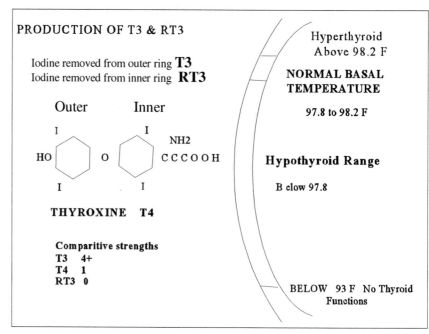

Figure 3

be as common as primary hypothyroidism.   In summary, the thyroid gland is similar to a propane tank that holds the fuel. The hypothalamus acts as the thermostat, while the pituitary is the control center making sure sufficient gas or T4 is delivered through the pipes, the blood vessels, to the furnace of the body cells, This constitutes the thyroid feed back cycle, the cycle that is checked out by the blood tests.

A **second control system** exists within the cells themselves, where T4 is converted to the more   active T3 and to RT3   (See Figure 3)[23] It is lack of attention to this control system that has caused a basic misunderstanding of thyroid function. The thyroxine molecule has two rings, each with two iodine atoms attached.. To produce T3, the body removes an iodine molecule from the outer ring of thyroxine or T4. The numbers three and four stand for the number of iodine atoms attached to the thyroid molecule. In other words, T3 has three iodine atoms in it while T4 has four iodine atoms in it. To produce RT3 an iodine is removed from the inner ring. Thus it

[22]Broda Barnes & Lawrence Galton; **Hypothyroidism the Unsuspected Illness**. Harper & Row, Publishers, 1976.

[23] Shimmel et. al.; **Thyroidal & Peripheral Production of Thyroid Hormones**. Annal of Internal Medicine 1979; 87 pp. 760-768.

also has three iodine atoms present. The angle between the two rings of thyroid hormone is affected by both the removal of the iodine and which ring it is taken from. This angle plays a critical role in the clinical effectiveness of the thyroid hormone. T3 has a ten times greater affinity for thyroid binding sites in the nucleus of the cell than T4 does and much of T3's increased activity may be due to this fact. RT3 has no metabolic activity whatsoever, though it can bind to thyroid binding sites, making these sites unavailable to the active T3 and T4. In chemistry this type of blockage is called competitive inhibition. So the rate of metabolism in the cell depends on the ratio of T4, T3, and RT3 in the cell. (There is a doctor in Florida who is calling the conversion of T4 to T3 by his own name, **Wilson's Syndrome.**[24])

CONVERSION OF T4 TO T3

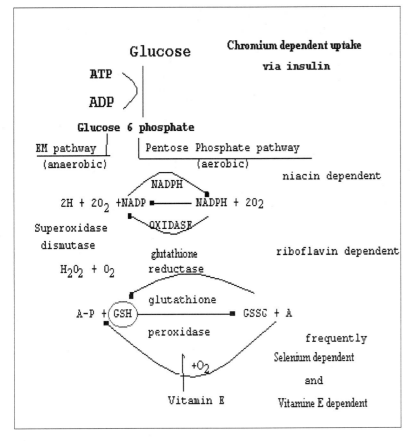

Figure 4

The enzyme that removes an iodine from T4 to convert it into T3 is a 5 DE-IODINASE Three different ones are known and are also responsible for converting T4 to RT3. Circumstantial evidence indicates the possibility of a fourth enzyme. The Type 1 de-iodinase is dependent on <u>sufficient amounts of GSH</u>. The diagram shows some of the minerals and vitamins that are important in supporting this process. Proper sugar metabolism, several B Vitamins, the antioxidant Vitamin E and antioxidant mineral selenium are all important. *Lack of glucose in the cell is the most important factor in decreasing Type I de-iodinase, thus decreasing T3 production.* In diabetics, glucose has a hard time entering the cells where this reaction takes place. Zinc and copper are also important in the enzyme activity. Current evidence indicates it is actually a cystein-selenium containing molecule.

---

[24] Dennis Wilson; **Wilson's Syndrome--The Miracle of Feeling Well**. Cornerstone Publishing Company, 1991.

This second control system has **two different divisions**. The first division is made up of the muscle and organs. Most of the brain, skin, and brown fat, the metabolically active fat in the body, make up the second division. These are structures that rise up from the ectoderm germ layer in a growing embryo. The first division comes from the germ layers that are termed endoderm and mesoderm. Though the chemistry may not mean anything to you, the important idea to grasp is that this Type I de-iodinase is sensitive to a lack of glucose in the cell, a lack of glucose shuts down the production of T3 and increases the production of RT3. (Figure 4) This is perhaps based on how acid the intercellular environment is which is indicated by the pH. The Western diet tends to produce excess acid. When a diet that alkalinizes the body is eaten, energy is often increased.. When there is a lack of glucose, a fermentation process starts in cells which produces lactic acid increasing the acidity of the cells. The usual metabolic cycle, the Krebs cycle, produces carbon dioxide. Likely this is a check which prevents a runaway metabolism during exercise. As lactic acid is , produced in exercise (produced by the cells when there is not enough oxygen) this mechanism shuts down metabolism in the cells so they do not become overheated. A body temperature more than 105 degrees F. is dangerous because disruption of cellular functions occurs and even cellular death.

The de-iodinase enzymes could be compared to valves which control the flow of oxygen to the furnace itself where the gas will be burned. If these valves are turned off, it doesn't matter how much gas is in the pipe line. Thyroid is not the fuel the body burns, but in some way thyroid hormone makes it possible for the body to burn its fuel, glucose, at higher rates. At this point, the analogy breaks down to some extent, for the thyroid is actually a catalyst for the oxygen or fuel supply and not oxygen or the fuel itself. It is known that anything that interferes with a proper fuel supply to the cells results in a decreased production of T3 and an increase in RT3---changes that are seen in many different illnesses. These changes produce a condition called the Euthyroid Sick Syndrome or Non-Thyroid Illness. Although T3 is always low in the Euthyroid Sick Syndrome, and thus metabolism is slowed, medicine has not regarded this condition as a thyroid illness. The reason is that the thyroid levels measured in the blood usually return to normal gradually when the illness is over. The possibility that chronic illness could keep T3 levels low is not considered. Though the exact process underlying Non-Thyroid Illness is still a matter of ongoing research, **the very fact that a T4 to T3 conversion problem exists in many separate conditions indicates that pure T4 preparations like Synthroid often are not converted to T3 as they should**

be.[25]   Recent research suggests that poor conversion is indeed a problem. As a result, T4 preparations are often not as effective clinically as the T3, T4 combinations found in desiccated thyroid preparations. (Paradoxically all types of hypothyroidism cause a **T4 to T3 conversion problem**, guaranteeing that primary hypothyroidism is not adequately treated by most doctors for there is an element of a T4 to T3 conversion problem present which is not taken into consideration.) This is partially due to the fact that thyroid hormone facilitates the entry of glucose into individual cells. It is likely that thyroid hormone facilitates its own entry into cells since these processes take energy. Thus it may be impossible to restore a true thyroid balance, a balance of the T4 and T3, at a cellular level with a T4 preparation alone for at times the conversion of T4 to T3 does not return to normal after an illness.

In the second system, *Type II de-iodinase*, a completely different enzyme, controls the conversion of T4 to T3. In this second system, the conversion of T4 to RT3 is controlled by a third de-iodinase, a third enzyme, *Type III*. Type II is not a selenium compound but the other two are.   Lack of selenium thus would tend to spare the brain at the expense of the rest of the body. This situation can occur in AIDS where the AIDS's virus uses up the body's stores of selenium in its own reproductive cycle.

There are other interesting differences in these de-iodinases. Type II enzyme activity is actually inhibited by high levels of T4---one of the reasons a tight control on T4 levels in the blood is important and likely one of the reasons depression and other mental problems can be seen in both hypothyroidism and hyperthyroidism. In both, the production of T3 in the brain cells may be decreased. It is also a reason that many individuals taking pure T4 preparations such as Synthroid don't feel as good---*they are suppressing the activity of their brains*. RT3 also inhibits the production of T3 in the brain and so may contribute to the malaise of illness. [26] RT3 levels in the blood are increased by the Thyroid Sick Syndrome brought on by all significant illness.

De-iodinases have important relationships to corticosteroids. In type I de-iodinase, cortisone **inhibits** the production of T3. However in type II, the production

_____

[25]Patricia Puglio; **Hypothyroidism, the Relation of Common Menstrual Disorders**. Womans Health Connection, 1997 II b pp. 2-3.

[26] Sing-yung Wu & Theo J. Visser; **Thyroid Hormone Metabolism-Molecular Biology.** CRC Press, 1994.

of T3 is greatly **enhanced**, increased a hundred fold in the laboratory experiments. This is the reason that adrenal hormones have such an impact on skin problems and on the functioning of the brain where Type II de-iodinase occurs. Steroids should be given a trial along with thyroid hormone if skin or mental problems are not clearing up on thyroid alone. A **third area of control** is in the

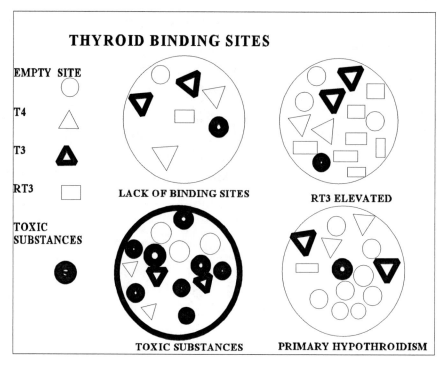

Figure 5

thyroid binding sites themselves. (Figure 5) When the binding sites are abnormal, one may develop what is called **thyroid resistance** ---the body does not respond to normal levels of thyroid hormone.[27] Current research seems to indicate that the thyroid binding sites in most cells are not saturated. In other words, even in a normal individual there are many extra binding sites available. It is the availability of these extra binding sites that makes hyperthyroidism possible. To a certain extent these extra binding sites can be taken up by estrogen and by toxic substancessuch as mercury. [28] At the least, extra estrogen and mercury contamination make it more likely that an individual will come down with the symptoms of hypothyroidism. The estrogen effect is likely the reason women complain of having hypothyroid symptoms four times more often than men. True thyroid resistance seems rare though, since it is not picked up by normal blood testing, the true incidence remains unknown. The rate of metabolism in the body is controlled by the amount of T3 produced and the adequacy of the thyroid binding sites. The basal temperature is an accurate reflection on what is taking place at a cellular level, and thus an essential indicator of proper thyroid functioning. For

[27] S. Raletoff; **Resistance to Thyroid Hormones.** Thyroid Today, Vol. 3 Oct. 1980.

[28] Hal. A. Huggins, DDS; **Its All In Your Head.** Life Science Press, 1990.

example, the urine test will not pick up thyroid resistance patients while the basal temperature will. It must be remembered that by interfering with the supply of glucose, low adrenal function will cause similar symptoms. One needs to remember that the temperature will be low in all the different types of hypothyroidism. Though a low metabolism may be obscured by fever or certain medications, this is not a significant clinical problem. *When a low basal temperature occurs, it always demands investigation since it usually indicates a problem with the thyroid-adrenal axis.* Just what action the thyroid has when it binds to the binding sites in the nucleus of the cells is not clearly understood. It is known that it plays a role in the transcription of information---in taking the genetic code and utilizing it to help synthesize or manufacture proteins. It is involved in the formation of enzymes and of neurotransmitters which send messages in the brain, for most of these are protein compounds. Thyroid is also involved in carbohydrate metabolism and in lipid metabolism. Every major function of the body is touched by thyroid. Some believe that the majority of these effects are mediated through the overall effect on metabolism. Though many of the effects can be explained by the control of metabolism alone, it does not explain all of them. Just the effects of thyroid hormone on the formation of enzymes could easily explain all of the roles played by thyroid since enzymes control all the chemical processes that take place in the body. The effects on lipid and carbohydrate metabolism may be secondary to thyroid's control of the production of key enzyme systems.

Once thyroid hormone has been formed, the body has to be able to get rid of it as well. There are a number of different pathways that the body uses to eliminate thyroid hormone from the cells. Both T4 & T3 are excreted in the urine by the kidneys and this forms the basis for the urine test for thyroid function. But a larger portion is processed by the liver. T3 can be further broken down to T2 and T1 in which only two, or one atoms of iodine respectively are present in the molecule. The iodine in the original thyroxine molecule is thus recycled, which is of particular importance when iodine intake is low. Some of the T3 and T4 is conjugated with a sulfate molecule in the liver and eliminated in the bile. In the intestines certain bacteria can strip the sulfate molecule off and the T3 and T4 produced may be reabsorbed by the body. This is the source of some of the T3 in the bloodstream, though most of the T3 present is released from the thyroid gland itself. Interestingly, in constipation, which is a feature of hypothyroidism, bacteria will have a greater chance of acting on the sulfate molecule, so a greater portion of the thyroid will be recycled. In hyperthyroidism stools are loose and diarrhea may occur so a larger portion of the thyroid will be eliminated from the body[29]. Also when adrenal function is low, diarrhea is apt to occur. This mechanism will help bring the ratio of thyroid to adrenal to a better balance.

Some research indicates that T2 may have regulatory functions in the body, but the research is still preliminary. The two rings which make up the thyroxine molecule or T4 can be split in two, releasing iodine which then may be used by the body to fight infections.

The control of thyroid hormones by the body is complex. Much more needs to be learned. But an elementary understanding of some of these basic processes is critical if one is to understand how thyroid functions in the body.

----

[29]

Sing-yung Wu, Theo J. Visser; **Thyroid hormone Metabolism-Molecular Biology**. CRC Press, 1994.

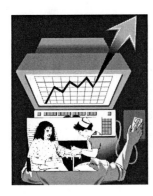

Chapter 6 **THYROID TESTS**

Lenny thought he had a thyroid problem but his blood tests did not show it. He had several blood tests run including the TSH and T4. It was not just that he was tired and sluggish. It was his lack of mental sharpness, his short term memory that was his biggest problem. He had tried supplements of various kinds. Though they helped some, his basic problem remained. It was difficult to carry on an ordinary conversation for suddenly he would forget what the conversation had been about. Rather than give an answer out of context, he would suddenly turn and walk away. His low basal metabolism and cluster of symptoms showed that he indeed had a hypothyroid condition that was not being picked up by the blood tests. On thyroid replacement therapy, his social gaffes stopped. His memory sharpened. He became normal in every way.

The enormous effect that thyroid had on metabolism was one of the first facts noted about the function of the thyroid gland and its hormones. Like in Lenny, it may have effects that are usually not attributed to a thyroid problem, such as his lack of social graces. But it was not long before doctors zeroed in on the metabolic effect of thyroid to devise the first test for thyroid function. The first test that was widely used was **the BMR** or **basal metabolic rate**. Interestingly enough, this test is still used occasionally to try to make sense out of a complex thyroid problem when the commonly used blood tests are not giving a clear answer. In checking the BMR, one is measuring metabolism by looking at the amount of oxygen consumed under resting conditions. The amount of oxygen consumed by the individual being tested has to be analyzed. This involves breathing into a mask or tube of some sort. Just having to breathe into a mechanical device causes problems in the test's reliability. How does one get the individual who is being tested to relax? And how does one know that the individual being tested is truly relaxed? If they are not relaxed, the basal metabolic rate is increased, sometimes in a dramatic fashion.

It does not take much to affect the basal metabolism rate. One cannot eat within five hours or the digestion of food will increase the rate. Vigorous exercise will leave the metabolic rate elevated for hours, so no exercise can be allowed for a full day. Then if the individual is sick, the measurements are meaningless, for any illness also will elevate the metabolic rate. But it was the difficulty in getting people to relax that led to the downfall of the BMR as the test of choice for diagnosing hypothyroid conditions. Dr. Broda Barnes tells of a student with obvious signs of hypothyroidism. On initial testing of his BMR, this obviously nervous student was running at plus 16 (On the BMR scale zero is normal and the scale runs from -40 to +40) A few jokes got the patient to relax and ten minutes later, the student was running a BMR score of minus 10. Other individuals tested had even more dramatic differences. So unless a doctor was sure the patient was relaxed when the BMR was done, unless he did the test himself, he could not know for sure if the results received from a clinical lab were reliable. This uncertainty was the reason the medical profession jumped onto the blood testing bandwagon when the first blood tests came out. The blood tests have been deceiving doctors ever since. The problems with the blood tests are just as real but not as widely appreciated as the problems with the BMR. **And they have been more detrimental to the public's health for they have led to a misunderstanding of hypothyroidism.**

PROBLEMATIC BLOOD TESTS

The first blood test used was the measurement of **protein bound iodine--- PBI**. Iodine and iodine containing compounds are transported by proteins in the blood stream. What was being measured was the T4, the T3 and the iodine that were being transported by these proteins. Though this test was used through the 1950's, a complex set of rules evolved around its use. The amount of protein in the blood is altered by a myriad of conditions and the protein levels in the blood had to be considered in interpreting the test, in deciding just how much thyroid hormone was available for use by the body. For example, pregnancy elevates the protein in the blood and malnutrition lowers it. The list of conditions affecting protein levels goes on and on. A simple act like taking an aspirin tablet changes the amount of iodine being carried by protein. And how often will the fact that the patient took an aspirin for a headache be missed because it does not seem important enough to the patient for him to mention? Eventually the medical profession decided the PBI was invalid and it was discarded. But the mischief had been done for as a result of that test, hypothyroidism was redefined. Up to that time at least 40% of the population was considered to be hypothyroid. On the basis of PBI testing the proportion of the population diagnosed as hypothyroid shrunk to less than 5%. The new blood tests that were added picked up the same population group, missing the majority of those whose metabolism was sluggish. Other conditions were postulated to try to explain the problems these individuals were having and their hypothyroidism remained undiagnosed.

In 1942 when the PBI test was just getting a strong hold on doctors, Broda Barnes added a refinement to basal metabolism testing. He came up with the **basal temperature test**. The temperature gives an accurate reflection of the body's metabolism. This test involves taking a ten minute temperature under the arm or axilla the first thing on awaking in the morning. Its first advantages was that the individual was relaxed on awaking. Even if a patient was nervous the body temperature did not have a chance to change significantly before the temperature was obtained. Since temperature is influenced by the menstrual cycle, Dr. Barnes found it was best to get the basal temperature in women starting the second day of their period and continuing for about three days. It makes no difference when men, young girls and women after menopause take their temperature. He decided on an axillary temperature because chronic sinus conditions are all too common in individuals with hypothyroidism. Dr. Barnes discovered that even a low grade, asymptomatic sinus infection could raise the oral temperature almost a degree. So the axillary temperature was more accurate---it just took more time to run. Taking it for ten minutes made it comparable to an oral temperature. The normal range should be 97.8° to 98.2° F.. He also found no difficulty diagnosing problem patients who could easily have been mis-diagnosed with the BMR. For example, in secondary hypothyroidism both thyroid and adrenal function are low. When individuals are low in adrenal function they can lose weight, run a fast pulse, even have a fine tremor---in other words, clinically look exactly like a hyperthyroid patient. If a patient was also nervous, as patients usually are, he would show a false elevation of the BMR. This type of individual showed up clearly as low thyroid on basal temperature testing. [30] **Unfortunately basal temperature testing never caught on.** Perhaps it was too simple. Perhaps it did not cost enough. Blood tests which were not nearly as accurate were used instead.

MORE PROBLEMATIC BLOOD TESTS

The next refinement in the blood tests was the **T4 blood test**. T4 testing ruled the roost for about twenty years through the 1970's. 99.9% of T4 and 99.7% of T3 are carried by proteins in the blood. Only the free or nonbound T4 and T3 molecules are considered active metabolically. Therefore, T4 testing shared many weaknesses with the PBI test. Nevertheless, it was an improvement, for the iodine carried by the blood stream was no longer measured. Other tests such as T3 uptake were soon added in an

---

[30]Broda O Barnes & Lawrence Galton; **Hypothyroidism the Unsuspected Illness**. Harper & Row Publishers, 1976.

attempt to gauge just how much T4 was bound to protein. More recently free, or non protein bound T4, is being measured by a more sophisticated blood test (rather than all the T4 in the blood), testing which is technically more difficult. This test is simply called the free T4 test.

Still, all these refinements in the testing miss the real problems in testing for the T4 levels. Some internists soon recognized that an overlap occurred between normal individuals, and individuals who were hypothyroid. So if a patient had the symptoms of low thyroid, they might give the patient thyroid hormone although his T4 level was in the low normal range. Unfortunately, the wisdom of this previous generation has been lost and thyroid is rarely given today when blood tests fall within the normal range. Dr. Broda Barnes checked out each blood test as it came into general use to try to gauge its accuracy. When the T4 test became popular, he ran this test on many of his patients---not just once a day but up to six times a day. He discovered he was getting *a different reading almost every time*. **Something was clearly wrong with the test**. Years earlier, when this test first became available, a researcher had canalized (inserted a catheter) into the thyroid veins of a few patients and had measured the T4 output directly from the thyroid gland. All these patients had normal T4 blood tests; normal range for most labs for the T4 test is 4.5 mcg to 12 mcg. Within this normal range there is a little less than a three-fold difference between the lowest normal value for the T4 and its highest value. He found that the actual output of the thyroid gland was varying ninety fold from the low level to the high level among these patients whose tests fell within the normal range. [31] These results, both the variability of results and the large difference in output in the normal range, indicate that the output of T4 is dynamic, not static, and likely varies throughout the day. Unless the output of thyroid over time is added to the equation, the results of T4 testing are totally inadequate.

An analogy will perhaps help us understand the problem. Walking by a mountain stream one notices that in some parts of the stream, there are deep pools. In other parts of the stream where the water is rushing swiftly the water is shallow. Yet the same amount of water is flowing past each part of the stream. What one is doing in T4 testing is lowering a stick into the water and measuring the depth of the stream. In one place the stream is three inches deep. In another place the stream is two feet deep. If one concluded that more water was flowing where the water was two feet deep, this conclusion would be wrong because the rate of flow at that point is not

---

[31]Leslie J. Degroot; **The Thyroid and Its Diseases**. Churchill Lingston, 1978.

being considered. In fact the same amount of water is flowing past both points. But how fast thyroid hormones are flowing into the cells is not considered in T 4 testing. The depth of the thyroid "stream" is being equated with how much water is flowing in the system. The amount of T4 produced by the body varies throughout the day in response to differing energy needs. T4 testing, to have any reliability as a diagnostic tool, must be measured over time. How important this factor is, is seen in some more recent information. The majority of thyroid hormone is carried by hemoglobin, not blood serum. Fully 95% of the thyroid hormone in the blood may be carried by hemoglobin in the red blood cells. The thyroid gland releases far more T3 than would be suspected from the blood tests. Much of the T 3 is carried by the red blood cells. T 3 flows into the cells much more rapidly than T 4. T 3 levels also remain low in the blood serum because it is taken up much more readily by the cells than is T4.

There are other pitfalls in T4 testing as well. For example, if one has had diagnostic tests using some of the iodine-containing radiological dyes, the residual iodine from the dyes can throw the results of T4 testing off for several months. [32]

	Thyroid/24 hrs	TSH	T4/T3 Urine/24hr	T3 produced	T4 blood
PATIENT # 1	300 mg	3.4 MCIU	256 mg	210 mg	8 mcg
PATIENT # 2	150 mg	3.4 MCIU	120 mg	105 mg	8 mcg

Table 3

Blood levels of TSH & T4 can be identical when very different amounts of T3 are produced.

Before leaving the T4 testing one last topic needs to be addressed. **It is possible for individuals to be hypothyroid and have elevated levels of T4.** This is sometimes seen in liver disease. The liver utilizes large amounts of thyroid. If liver cells are not able to use all the thyroid brought to them by the blood stream, the thyroid backs up and the blood levels of thyroid hormone rise, similar to when a stream is

---

[32]Lewis E. Baverman; **Warner & Ingbars The Thyroid.** Lippincott & Ravens Publishers, 1996.

dammed. Since T4 levels in the blood are high, TSH will be low. In other words these individuals have the classic blood results seen in hyperthyroidism. The basal metabolism and their symptom clusters will clearly show that these individuals with chronic liver disease are frequently hypothyroid.

THE INADEQUACY OF THE TSH

The **TSH test** took center stage in the eighties and still holds its position as the premier test for diagnosing thyroid problems, although cracks are starting to show in some of the original foundational assumptions. The TSH first gained its reputation in a head-to-head confrontation with T4 testing in known, primary hypothyroid patients in the late seventies. It did a better job than the T4 test in this setting likely because the TSH was responding to the levels of both T4 and T3 in the cells of the hypothalamus. Soon afterwards, more accurate tests for measuring TSH were developed which were able to measure smaller amounts of TSH, so the status of the TSH test was elevated, almost to godhood. The first new generation of tests enabled the detection of TSH levels ten times smaller than those observed by the earlier tests. Recently, a third generation of the tests increased this sensitivity another ten-fold. No clinical usefulness will result from tests that will pick up even smaller amounts of TSH than the current tests are able to do. [33]

It has always been known that the TSH test had at least one primary defect. It did not pick up secondary or tertiary hypothyroidism. When the pituitary or hypothalamus is not working properly, the TSH comes back either normal or more often low, under 0.3 MCIU in most labs. It will come back low because the pituitary is producing such a small amount of TSH that the TSH does not signal the thyroid gland to put out sufficient thyroid (T4 or thyroxin). It can come back normal since at times, though sufficient TSH is being produced, this TSH is defective in quality and does not signal the thyroid to put out enough thyroid hormone either. One cannot evaluate a patient adequately if he has hypothyroid symptoms with just a TSH test, since it will miss secondary thyroid patients. A normal test does not mean the patient is normal. Some doctors indicate that at a minimum a T4 test should also be run. But often today the TSH is being utilized as a screening test for thyroid problems without any other thyroid tests.

---

[33]Ibid

This inability to pick up secondary hypothyroid patients, though just one of many problems the TSH test has, may be more significant than usually realized. Some have considered secondary hypothyroidism as unimportant since its incidence is often reported as less than 1 percent of the hypothyroid population. Other reports say that a more accurate figure is closer to 5%. Both reports are likely wrong---mild problems with the pituitary-hypothalamic axis are far more common than suspected. Dr. Kellman ran a test called the **thyrotrophic hormone stimulation test** in chronic fatigue patients, a test designed to investigate how well the pituitary is functioning in thyroid disease. In this test the patient is given a bolus, an injection, of THR, thyrotrophic releasing hormone and the TSH response is measured to this stimulation. Normally TSH will increase to a level of 30 MCIU. These individuals had already shown TSH and T4 test levels within the normal range. He found that 40% of these individuals showed problems with their anterior pituitary gland with this test. Then Dr. Levin ran tests in women who were diagnosed as having fibromyalgia. 10% of these women showed primary hypothyroidism by TSH & T4 testing. He then did the thyrotrophic stimulation test and found another 50% showed definite abnormalities in pituitary function. He placed the remaining patients who showed no abnormalities at all, according to their blood tests, on thyroid. He discovered that thyroid was just as important in helping these patients recover from their symptoms of fibromyalgia as those who showed they had a problem on the blood tests. Another type of hypothyroid problem was apparently involved in these individuals---a thyroid problem within the cells themselves. Though secondary hypothyroidism will show up on special blood tests, these other problems do not on the currently used tests, so they are not even considered by the medical profession at large. Actually a low T4 along with a low TSH usually indicates an element of secondary hypothyroidism but the general reaction of the medical profession is that the individual's thyroid level is too high and if on replacement therapy, their thyroid dosage is decreased.

How common is secondary hypothyroidism? No one really knows. In general, doctors do not test for secondary hypothyroidism, so this condition is not being found. As individuals grow older, after age sixty nearly 5 % may show was is called subclinical hyperthyroidism. These individuals have normal T4 levels on their blood tests, but show suppressed TSH levels, often so low that it can't be measured, just as one sees in true hyperthyroidism. When followed over time the TSH test returns to normal in about one quarter of these individuals. Only about 2% or less of them go on to become truly hyperthyroid. 'Hyperthyroidism' (individuals diagnosed as hyperthyroid who may not be) in the elderly tends to be subtle, 48 % exhibiting some signs more typical of hypothyroidism. These patients are treated as hyperthyroid and have the output of their thyroid gland decreased by medication or radioactive iodine due to the increase in atrial fibrillation seen in this population. I suspect many of these subclinical hyperthyroid patients and 'hyperthyroid' patients would be found to have an abnormality of the pituitary if adequately tested and are in reality mild secondary hypothyroid patients. The adrenal insufficiency in these patients may underlie the atrial fibrillation that is being seen.

Even though one rules out secondary hypothyroidism, the TSH test still has substantial problems. Among the more minor problems, a few individuals fall outside the normal range, as was mentioned in the population over age sixty. Their tests show levels either too high or too low when in reality their hormone production may be just right. Also, all hormones have circadian rhythms. This is certainly true of TSH. TSH levels are highest at night and lowest around 11 o'clock in the morning. In fact if TSH levels are tested at night they will usually be found to be slightly high. So an individual should have the TSH taken the same time each day. Adding to the problem, almost all endocrine glands put their hormones out in spurts. Again this is true of TSH. So the level one gets in measuring TSH depends on where one catches a spurt when the blood is drawn. A more significant problem is the problem of Non Thyroid Illness or the Euthyroid Sick Syndrome. Any acute illness, if it is severe enough, will throw TSH testing off. Usually the TSH will be elevated, though it can be low as well. There is no way to predict how the levels will be affected. After an acute illness it may take four months for the TSH to return to values seen prior to the illness. Acute psychiatric illness has the same effect as other illnesses. And certain types of chronic illness, particularly chronic liver disease, interfere with thyroid testing, making the TSH unreliable when these conditions are present.

THE PROBLEM OF THE TSH SET POINT

The biggest problem with TSH testing lies in a different realm altogether. Part of the usefulness of the TSH testing is that it has a magnifying effect, magnifying the changes in T4 levels. Double one's T4, and the TSH increases eighty times. This is a constant relationship. The TSH thus makes it easier to see small changes in T4. The problem is that all individuals words, one individual may have a TSH of 0.3 MCIU and a corresponding T4 lev have their own unique relationships between their TSH and their T4 levels. In other el of 8 mcg. Another individual may have a TSH of 4.5 MCIU and a corresponding T4 level of 8 mcg.. If the first individual (TSH 0.3 MCIU) were to develop primary hypothyroidism and were treated to bring the TSH back into a normal range, just bringing this individual back to a normal TSH level of 4.5 MCIU would be totally inadequate. He would need sufficient replacement therapy to bring his TSH down to 0.3 in order to function normally. Some endocrinologists are starting to use clinical symptoms to determine what the TSH target level should be for each individual. Why not just use the clinical symptoms to start with in light of the other problems that can cause variations in TSH levels? The very fact that older patients tend to have low TSH tests indicates that the proper TSH levels may change with time, likely as the efficiency of the anterior pituitary gland decreases. Yes, one often can confirm a diagnosis of primary hypothyroidism with the TSH test. But it cannot be used as an adequate guide for replacement therapy for all of the above reasons.

TSH LEVELS	T4 Levels	TSH after becoming Hypothyroid	New T4 Levels	TSH replacement therapy	T4 levels on therapy
0.1 MCIU	8 mcg	20 MCIU	3.2 mcg	4.5 MCIU	4.5 mcg
0.3 MCIU	8 mcg	20 MCIU	4.8 mcg	4.5 MCIU	5.5 mcg
1 MCIU	8 mcg	20 MCIU	6 mcg	4.5 MCIU	7.6 mcg
4.5 MCIU	8 mcg	20 MCIU	7.6 mcg	4.5 MCIU	8 mcg

Table 4   **Relationship between T4 & TSH**

Another problem that confounds the blood tests is the fact that a substantial number of patients develop auto-antibodies to thyroid, somewhere around fifteen to twenty percent of individuals in many series. Some authorities believe it is important to test patients for this condition. If auto-antibodies are present, they believe it renders other thyroid testing invalid. They believe that if these antibodies are present, they may destroy the T4 or T3 one is measuring before the body can utilize it. Therefore seeing a normal T4 level on the blood tests has little meaning under these circumstances. One has no idea how much of the T4 or T3 that is being measured has any clinical effect.

Perhaps the problems with the blood tests can be summarized by the experiences of Broda Barnes. He ran a series of blood tests on thirty new hypothyroid patients---individuals who were symptomatic and showed the need for thyroid when their basal metabolism was checked. He then ran as controls a group of patients that were fully treated with thyroid for their hypothyroidism, patients who had become completely symptom free. There was no difference in results for these two groups of patients. **The blood tests on the treated patients and the untreated patients came back almost exactly the same.** [34]

If there is a **blood test that may eventually become the true 'gold standard'** for thyroid testing, it will likely be the blood test for free T3. As mentioned in the chapter on metabolism, it is the T3 that is the active thyroid hormone.   When T3 is produced in the cells, some leaks out into the blood stream. Since it is not present in very large quantities, it has been ignored by the medical profession.   But the amounts present in the blood seem to correlate quite well with the basal temperature. Those who have started using this test find that a level of 320 pic. grams to 340 pic. grams/liter appears to correlate well with normal thyroid functions. In the literature, the range given for normal is too broad and this has curtailed the usefulness of this test up to now because those who are low thyroid are included with those who have normal thyroid function.

Down through the years doctors have used a variety of other tests as an indicator of thyroid function.   One of these was cholesterol---a high cholesterol was used to indicate a hypothyroid problem.   Since hypothyroidism can also cause very low cholesterol levels, cholesterol levels provide little help beyond suggesting a thyroid problem may exist if cholesterol levels are abnormal. Whether too low or too high, certainly cholesterol tests alone should not be relied on to diagnose thyroid disease. Others have used the ankle reflex as an indicator of hypothyroidism. A slow relaxation phase on testing this reflex is the indicator. But without special equipment, it is difficult to quantify this reaction accurately enough for the test to be a true help. Again, any sluggish reflex is suggestive of a hypothyroid problem. A simple EKG can be suggestive as well. Low voltage on an EKG is usually indicative of a hypothyroid problem.

The newest test for thyroid problems is **the twenty four hour urine test for T3 and T4.**   It is a useful test, because its results usually parallel the basal temperature or metabolism. Various adrenal hormones are also measured in the urine also giving some insight into the adrenal function in the individuals tested. This test meets the need

---

[34]Broda O Barnes & Lawrence Galton; **Hypothyroidism the Unsuspected Illness.** Harper & Row Publishers,   1976.

for adding time to T4 and T3 measurements and gives some indication of what portion of lowered basal temperature, a lowered metabolism is due to the thyroid condition and how much is due to an inadequate adrenal function. This test too can be misleading at times, so in the final analysis it is important to evaluate each individual clinically. But this test is quite expensive, partly because of the number of adrenal hormones evaluated. At present it is only being run by one laboratory in Europe, thus, it is not generally available. Also it often takes a couple of months to get results back. If this type of testing were in general use, the cost would come down to reasonable levels.

No test has replaced the effectiveness and simplicity of the basal temperature test. And this test is free. All it costs is a little time and the price of a mercury thermometer. The basal temperature should always be considered in any thyroid problem---it will prevent doctors from making tragic mistakes.

Perhaps the problem of thyroid testing will be seen more clearly if an analogy is used to illustrate the current status of thyroid testing. Since the thyroid provides the body with its heating system (regulates its metabolism) we will again compare it to a furnace in one's home. The patient, the owner of the house, his own body, calls and says:

"Hey, doc, Something must be wrong with my heating system. My house is cold."

"I'll come right out and check the problem for you." The next day the doctor says, "I've good news for you. I used a great test we doctors call the TSH test and I can assure you, you have pipelines (the veins & arteries) that have plenty of gas (T4) in them. You shouldn't be having any problem at all."

"But my house is still cold. Aren't there any other tests you can run?"

"Well, yes. Sometimes we doctors will run other tests. And if you insist I will run some more."

The next day he again calls saying, "I have more good news for you. I ran a free T4 test and it too was normal. I can assure you the pipelines in your house are large enough to carry an adequate supply of fuel (the T4) to your furnace. And because you were so concerned I also ran a Thyrotrophic Stimulation Test. I even checked out your thermostat (the hypothalamus and pituitary). And though there may be a tiny abnormality in its function, I don't think it should be giving you any significant problem."

"But Doc, my house is still cold. Isn't there any test left that you can run."

"Well, yes there is one." The next day he again calls and says, "I have more good news. I ran tests for auto antibodies. And I can tell you, you have no water mixed in with your gas. Your whole system is perfectly normal."

"But Doc, didn't you check my furnace to see if the fire was burning properly there?"

"What, check your furnace? That testing is not included in our standards. Why don't you go and see your friendly psychiatrist if you still think that you are cold?"

Sadly this is exactly what is happening to far too many patients today. The first thing one needs to do is check the fire in the furnace---check the basal temperature. The fire must be hot enough, the rate of metabolism *must* be examined.

Chapter 7   The relationship of Thyroid and Adrenal
Hormones

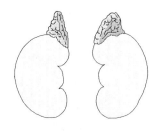

Adrenal Glands

Alice was in her early seventies and had been a prisoner in her own house for thirteen years. Diarrhea imprisoned her. It was not just that she had frequent stools throughout the day; she had no idea when the bowel movements were going to happen. She did not feel them coming on. Any social life was impossible. She could not shop. She could not go to church nor enjoy all the other activities she loved doing. She also had the coldness and tiredness seen with a hypothyroid condition. But hypothyroidism alone usually causes constipation, not diarrhea. Poor Alice! Both her thyroid and adrenal function were off. On replacement therapy for both her thyroid and adrenal glands she gradually improved. The diarrhea slowed, then stopped. She regained sensation in her bowels and actually knew when she needed to go to the bathroom. She could get out of her home again at last. Fifteen years later, following hip fractures and other medical problems, she is still able to get out, though she is not as spry as she used to be. The combination of thyroid and prednisone restored her to a nearly normal life.

Like in Alice, supporting the adrenal function is often critical in restoring an individual to good health. The adrenal glands are perched on top of the kidneys. The functions of the thyroid are intertwined with the functioning of the adrenal hormones, particularly with the glucocorticoids at many different levels, in different portions of their respective metabolic pathways. The many different areas where they interconnect with each other have obscured the most important relationship between these two classes of hormones---this particular relationship is not even discussed in recent textbooks on thyroid function. This relationship is their **mutual control over metabolism**---the thyroid by regulating the rate at which glucose, the body's main fuel is burned; the adrenal by regulating the availability of that same fuel. The adrenal hormones, the glucocorticoids,[35] control the release of glucose from several different areas. The first is from its storage as glycogen in the liver thus providing glucose which is immediately available for energy production. Next fat deposits are utilized to provide the glucose needed for fuel. Other hormones such as glucagon are active in this process. Fat stores are the main source utilized to provide for the long term energy needs of the body. In a pinch, body proteins such as the ones in muscle are broken down to provide the needed glucose.. Like thyroid, the glucocorticoids work in the

---

[35] William McK Jeffries; **Safe Uses of Cortisone**. 1994

nucleus of the cell to enhance the transcription of certain proteins that have effects elsewhere in the body. So the thyroid and adrenal must work together to provide the body with sufficient energy to meet the challenges that it faces. When the body is under stress it usually needs extra energy, so the adrenal glands start supplying extra glucose, preparing the body to meet the crisis, no matter what it is. When bacterial hordes invade the body, for example, this invasion signals the adrenal to provide extra glucose, mobilizing this resource to be available to help fight off the invaders. The thyroid then has to handle the burning of this extra fuel which the adrenal provides. If insufficient thyroid is available, the body will have a hard time meeting the stressful challenges it faces. The differences in providing the glucose (adrenal function) and in overseeing its utilization (thyroid function) lead to different patterns depending on whether the thyroid deficiency is primary (is the greater problem) or the adrenal deficiency is primary, (as great or greater than the thyroid deficiency). For example, if the adrenal reserves are inadequate, the body may be able to garner the energy needed for a short lived "crisis", for the energy expenditure by the body has to be greater than normal only for a short period of time. But when the readily available reserves of glucose are gone it can take hours for the glucocorticoids to release adequate amounts of glucose from the body's long term stores to bring ready reserves of fuel back to what the body needs to have on hand, so frequently a long recovery phase occurs after any stress when adrenal function is inadequate. Individuals with inadequate adrenal function crash and may have to rest for a couple of days before their energy levels return to normal functioning levels. So low adrenal individuals frequently become exhausted after they have had to do more than slow paced activities. This prolonged need for recovery often leaves these individuals tired when they wake up in the morning, while pure hypothyroid patients are more apt to have good energy on awaking but tire as they face the tasks of the day. Again this interrelationship in providing the body with its energy means that a deficiency in either thyroid or the glucocorticoids produces symptoms that mimic each other's deficiencies. Both will result in a low body temperature, for example. These relationships are discussed further in the chapter on the symptoms and signs of hypothyroidism.

Let's discuss some of the other key interrelationships between the thyroid and the adrenal. When hydrocortisone was first used clinically, it was used in the treatment of rheumatoid arthritis. How much hydrocortisone was produced by the body, by the adrenal glands, was not known at that time, but a dosage of 300 mg a day was chosen because at this dose almost all the symptoms of the rheumatoid arthritis would vanish in two or three days. This is roughly three times the amount of steroid that the body produces even under conditions of extreme stress. It was not long before these rheumatoid arthritis patients were developing all the classic signs of a steroid overdose. Out of the research done to understand these steroid side effects, it was discovered that high pharmacologic doses of steroids shut down thyroid function almost completely. Too often the clinical importance of this fact has not been appreciated. Large doses of adrenal hormones will make an individual hypothyroid. Unfortunately, even when large doses of steroids are given over long periods of time, doctors are not supporting thyroid function. This is a mistake. Many of the side effects of the steroids would be minimized (and actually much smaller dosages of the steroids could be given) if thyroid was added to the regimen. The other misunderstanding that arose in the medical profession was that of the therapeutic effects of physiologic doses of steroids, amounts of steroids equal to or less than the normal range of hormones actually put out by the normal human body. Because large doses of steroids produce so many horrible side effects, it was assumed that smaller doses would as well, only it would take longer for these side effects to show up. This is not true. Physiologic doses of steroids do not cause side effects if these doses are balanced with thyroid hormones. Often the effects of low dose steroids are the opposite of the effects seen with high or pharmacologic doses. For example, physiologic doses of steroids strengthen the immune system, rather than weaken it like large doses do.

The adrenal glucocorticoids given in large doses suppress TSH levels. It is the TSH as mentioned earlier which signals the thyroid to release its hormones. This is the primary reason the thyroid shuts down when large doses of steroids are given. But the steroids play other roles as well. The glucocorticoids have a direct effect on the release of thyroid hormone from the thyroid gland, though it is likely of minor importance. But the impact these steroids have on the de-iodinase enzymes, enzymes that control the conversion of T4, the transport thyroid hormone, to its much more active T3 form in the cells is crucial. There are two major divisions in the de-iodinase hormones and each division handles the conversion of T4 to T3 differently. [36] The steroids suppress one division and greatly enhance the other. In the developing embryo, three different germ layers soon can be distinguished: the ectoderm, endoderm and mesoderm. The ectoderm layer develops into the nervous system, the brain and the skin. These tissues arising from the ectoderm, along with a substance called brown fat, share one control system while the rest of the body shares the other control system. The organs and the

---

[36]Sing-yung Wu & Theo J. Visser; **Thyroid Hormone Metabolism-Molecular Biology.** CRC Press, 1994.

muscles, thus the portion of the body where the majority of metabolism takes place, is controlled by the type I de-iodinase. The brain and skin are controlled by the Type II de-iodinase. Most of the metabolism of the body is slowed down by the glucocorticoids because, by far the larger mass of the body is controlled by the type 1 de-iodinase. On the other hand any condition that affects the skin or the brain may be improved by the addition of steroids because they greatly enhance the activity of type 2 de-iodinase. This includes depression and other emotional difficulties. The steroids can even help weight problems in some individuals. And that goes back to the brown fat which was mentioned. Brown fat is metabolically active fat. The more active brown fat an individual has, the more calories that individual burns. Activating brown fat will help control weight. And low dose steroids can help activate brown fat.

It is the balance between thyroid and adrenal that is important. I suspect that most of the problems seen in hyperthyroidism are due to a relative adrenal insufficiency. The reason for this statement is that in infants both thyroid and adrenal levels are much higher than in the adult. For example, thyroid levels run around fifteen times higher while pregnenolone, the first of the adrenal hormones has levels that are twenty times higher than seen in adulthood. Yet these infants are in perfect metabolic balance---their high blood levels of thyroid, much higher than in adult hyperthyroidism are not giving them any problems for the thyroid is balanced with more adrenal hormone.

One additional relationship should be mentioned briefly. In 1989 researchers were surprised to find that there was a close structural relationship of the binding sites of thyroid hormone in the nucleus of the cell to the binding sites for steroids. Both thyroid hormones and steroid hormones have their binding sites in the nucleus of cells and produce their functions through attachment to these sites. Recently estrogen, also a hormone produced by the adrenal gland, has been found to bind to thyroid binding sites with ease. Excess estrogen thus decreases thyroid function by tying up its binding sites. Progesterone, an adrenal hormone but also a female sex hormone, counters the effects of estrogen excess, perhaps blocking its attachment to thyroid binding sites. Progesterone is known to enhance thyroid function. More of this relationship will be discussed in the chapter on problems unique to women.

Both thyroid and adrenal hormones are controlled by the pituitary and the hypothalamus. When problems exist in the functioning of either the hypothalamus or the pituitary, both the thyroid and adrenal glands are usually affected. Both may have an inadequate output, and both the thyroid and adrenal glands may need support in order to restore an individual with a pituitary problem to health. Just having a hypothyroid problem will often result in sluggish adrenal function. But this sluggishness will correct itself with time. And though initial adrenal support is often helpful, these individuals will eventually do well without any adrenal support. This is not true when the problem is in the control centers in the brain. These individuals will always need adrenal support along with the thyroid. Interestingly, at times the initial symptoms of individuals who have secondary hypothyroidism may be milder than those seen in primary hypothyroidism since the thyroid and adrenal are in better balance. But more often their symptoms are more severe and they will have a much greater variety of symptoms, often with all parts of the body involved.

The important point to remember is that if a patient with low adrenal function is put on thyroid replacement without giving any adrenal support, he can be thrown into shock from adrenal insufficiency. [37] The reason for this is that thyroid increases the metabolic activity of the adrenal hormones. In other words, the body gets rid of the supply of adrenal hormones it has on hand more quickly, leaving the individual with an inadequate amount of adrenal hormones in reserve to take care of the needs of the body. Adrenal hormones, particularly the mineral corticoids, control blood volume through their effect on water and salt (sodium) metabolism. With insufficient adrenal hormones, the blood volume decreases and becomes insufficient to maintain blood pressure so the individuals are liable to go into shock. People with low adrenal function frequently require additional salt in their diet to keep their blood volume up. Recently, inadequate circulating blood volume has been found to be a cause of mitral valve prolapse and many of its symptoms, a condition seen in about 10% of the population.

Some of the impact of hypothyroidism on the adrenal gland is mediated through the thyroid hormone's effects on cholesterol. All adrenal hormones are manufactured from cholesterol. When individuals are hypothyroid two different patterns are seen regarding cholesterol. In some individuals the cholesterol levels are quite low. However, in most individuals cholesterol levels are elevated. Though poor absorption of dietary cholesterol may play a part when cholesterol levels are low, the liver is likely more responsible. The liver manufactures two thirds of an individual's cholesterol, only one third comes from the diet. When individuals have a low cholesterol it is likely

---

[37] Physicians Desk Reference, 1997.

the liver is not manufacturing sufficient quantities of cholesterol because the liver's own function is sluggish due to hypothyroidism. When insufficient amounts of cholesterol are formed, enough cholesterol to manufacture the needed adrenal hormones may not be available.

But what about those with high cholesterol levels? These levels may be high simply because the body is not using the cholesterol properly. In other words, the body may be having a hard time manufacturing adequate amounts of steroids from the cholesterol. (Cholesterol does have other important functions, providing, for example, most of the insulation for the nervous system and brain). It is known that in hypothyroidism the production of adrenal hormones is sluggish---in fact, when hypothyroidism is severe, the adrenal gland can actually atrophy. Usually the body still has enough adrenal reserve to meet any ordinary crisis it might face. But these individuals may develop symptoms which suggest the adrenal is having a hard time keeping up when under stress. Of course there may be problems with any of the many enzymes that control individual steps of adrenal function. The adrenal gland produces dozens of different steroids when the various intermediary steps are counted. Actually most of these compounds are active. Thus many different clinical pictures are possible. But, in general, after individuals have been on thyroid for some time the underlying problem with cholesterol metabolism is corrected and they no longer need to continue adrenal support. It also means that different types of adrenal support may be important. The female hormones, both estrogen and progesterone, may be essential in restoring normal function in an individual. Most individuals started on thyroid will require less than six months of adrenal support. These individuals will be able to go off their low dose steroids without tapering the dosage. If they cannot, this indicates they still need adrenal support. Current research is showing that in patients with problems in which the steroids have been traditionally used such as allergies, inflammatory arthritis, and connective tissue disorders, there is an underlying mild adrenal insufficiency.[38] It is beneficial to add adrenal support to such individuals when placing them on thyroid, for the adrenal gland will be weak.

The functions of the adrenal and the thyroid are so closely intertwined it is imperative to consider both systems when treating an individual for either hypothyroidism or for adrenal insufficiency. If the treating physician does not do

---

[38]William McK. Jeferies MD; **Mild Adrenocortical Deficiency, Chronic Allergies**. Medical Hypotheses, May, 1994; 42 pp. 193-189.

so, he or she will greatly increase the problems faced in taking care of this individual. Nearly half of hypothyroid patients will benefit from temporary adrenal support. Perhaps five percent will need some adrenal support on a permanent basis. Being aware of this relationship will minimize the problems encountered in thyroid replacement therapy.

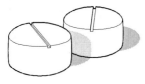

Chapter 8   Thyroid & Adrenal Preparations

Mary had been on Synthroid for years, having been diagnosed as having a primary hypothyroid condition. She had felt better since starting the Synthroid, but her health was not good. Her skin was still dry. She frequently napped in the afternoon. If she did not, she would have a hard time finishing her evening chores. She was mildly depressed. Her short-term memory had deserted her. She was not sleeping well at night. Her health was getting worse. She was switched to natural desiccated thyroid and the dosage was gradually increased to three grains. All her symptoms went away.

The kind of thyroid one takes can play an important role in the recovery from the symptoms of hypothyroidism, as Mary found out, by switching to a natural thyroid hormone, a product which contains both T3 & T4. There are some who are saying that T4 should not be called the thyroid hormone, which it often is. That designation should be given to T3, for in some cells, those from ectoderm, T4 decreases rather than increases function. This chapter deals with the different preparations which are available for supporting thyroid and adrenal function.

Thyroid Hormones

Thyroid hormones were first used for replacement therapy in the United States starting in about 1883. These first preparations were crude and many of them did not have much thyroid activity. Actually, their use resulted in a wrong clinical impression as to thyroid's effectiveness in various clinical conditions. The quality of these desiccated products rapidly improved. The term "desiccated" refers to the fact that the water has been removed from the product. Glandular tissue, like the rest of the body, starts out with 70% of weight being due to water. The original replacement products, like the desiccated products available today, came from either pork or bovine thyroid glands. These glands were frozen, ground up and dehydrated by removing the water content, usually under vacuum, so the active thyroid hormone was not damaged. Acetone was then used to purify the thyroid powder. Inert ingredients were then added to give bulk and to standardize the strength of the powder which was then compressed into pills. Eventually the standard was adopted of using the amount of iodine present in the preparation to indicate its strength. This is still the only standard that the FDA has adopted for the standardization of desiccated thyroid products, but it is not an adequate one. (Since the desiccated thyroid preparations preexisted the FDA and were brought in as is, there is a sense in which they are outside the regulations of the FDA.) When iodine content is the only criteria used to determine the strength of desiccated thyroid preparations, it is now well known that these preparations can vary four fold in potency. So one cannot trust the strength of preparations standardized by iodine content alone. Some of the crude, generic desiccated thyroid preparations only use the iodine content as a guide to their strength.[39] As a result these generic desiccated thyroid preparations will not give a patient consistently potent therapy. This weakness of some generic preparations has been exploited by the makers of synthetic thyroid. The often heard claim is that desiccated thyroid preparations are not to be trusted; they vary in potency. It is not true of the good name brands of desiccated thyroid. The best known of these is Armour Thyroid. The makers of Armour Thyroid introduced a double standardization process in their product line. A biological assay was added to the assay of iodine content. In other words the strength of the product is determined in living systems, in addition to the iodine content for each batch that is produced. Dr. Broda Barnes was involved in checking out the reliability of the Armour Thyroid. He not only found that it was consistent from batch to batch but that it retained its potency for considerable periods of time---for at least five years. The strength of the desiccated thyroid products is often expressed in grains. One grain equals 60 mg of thyroid. Desiccated thyroid is available in a number of different strengths----1/4 gr., ½ gr., 3/4 gr. , 1 gr., 1 ½ gr. , 2 gr., 3 gr., 4 gr., and 5 gr. tablets. The bulk of desiccated thyroid is made up of T4. A bit over a quarter of the tablet is T3, and then a small amount of T2 and other thyroid related products are also present. Not surprisingly the thyroid gland actually releases T4 and T3 in roughly the same proportions as found in the gland. The blood tests just don't reflect what the gland is actually doing. In taking natural thyroid one is getting what the body puts out. Various inert ingredients are added to the tablet to provide stability and bulk. Armour Thyroid has a small amount of corn syrup and lactose, or milk sugar, as part of the inert ingredients.

Around 1995 Armour Thyroid changed some of the inert ingredients in their preparation. It is the clinical impression of some of the doctors using this new formulation that it may not be absorbed quite as well as the original Armour Thyroid, so higher doses may be needed. Or the tablet may need to be chewed. On average only about half of the thyroid in a preparation is absorbed by the body. Changing the inert ingredients can change this absorption. For example, those who got by with three

---

[39] **Merck Manual,** 1979.

grains of thyroid before now often do better on four grains of Armour Thyroid.

The usual starting dose of desiccated thyroid in an adult is one grain. In some large individuals it may be appropriate to start at a dosage level of two grains. The starting dose for a child should be ½ gr. and for an infant 1/4 gr. It takes at least five grains of thyroid to suppress a thyroid gland fully in a normal adult. The most common dosage needed to rid most adults of all hypothyroid symptoms is three grains. The amounts of thyroid needed in children are relatively greater. When congenital hypothyroidism is picked up in an infant, a dosage of 12-16 Ug./kg body weight is often recommended.[40] The requirements gradually decrease through childhood, although at age eight to ten years the requirements may still be at 3 Ug./kg, twice the adult requirement of 1.5 Ug./ kg. After two weeks on a given dose, the blood level stabilizes. In reality there is a minute increase in the blood levels for up to three months but it has no clinical significance after two weeks. For this reason dosage is usually increased at intervals of a month, giving about two weeks to assess clinical symptoms for each size dose. Clinical symptoms remain the best indicator of adequate dosages. Temperature is an important check in that if too much thyroid is given, dosages that will put the individual into a hyperthyroid range, this will show up in his temperature in the two-week time frame. There is a seasonal variation in thyroid needs. Individuals need a little more in the winter, and a little less in the summer when the weather is warm. For many this difference is not clinically important. But for some this adjustment is helpful.

Two other excellent desiccated thyroid products are put out by Jones Pharmaceuticals. Westhroid is similar to Armour Thyroid and is cheaper. But since it is not as widely known it is harder to find at most drug stores. Nature-Throid has the advantage of not having any milk or corn products in its inert fillers. As a result those with allergy problems may do better on this preparation. Both Westhroid and Nature-Throid undergo a double standardization in their manufacture and are consistent from batch to batch.

Various simple over the counter thyroid glandular products are also available. The problem with these products is that some of them have most of the active thyroid removed. Others do not. So no general recommendations can be give for these

---

[40] Gerald N. Burrow, Jean Dussault, et al.; **Neonatal Thyroid Screening**, Raven Press New York, 1980.

products other than it one wishes to use them, some of them will work well if increased gradually until symptoms are controlled. Only mild thyroid conditions will be improved if the active thyroid hormones have been removed. Often it will say on the label that thyroxin, active thyroid hormone has been removed.

In the 1960's the synthetic thyroids were introduced. These had the theoretical advantage of being more consistent in potency from batch to batch, though this consistency has not proved true in practice. It also was easier to interpret thyroid blood tests on the synthetic thyroid hormones since one only had to measure the T4 in the blood. Synthroid is the leading brand name among these products. Synthroid is a pure T4 preparation. Since T4 is converted to T3 in peripheral tissue of the body, it was assumed that giving synthroid would be equivalent to giving the desiccated products, unfortunately this is not true. This assumption was never tested in clinical studies and the synthetic products were never formally approved by the FDA. In many patients taking Synthroid only a partial portion of the usual conversion of the T4 to T3 occurs at best. Pure T4 can act as an anti-hormone in the brain and thyroid levels there are actually decreased by taking Synthroid. Therefore, many patients who take Synthroid do not get the same clinical response to it as they do to the desiccated thyroid products. Even when patients feel good on the synthetic products, they are not getting all the benefits they should.

More recently, additional problems have come to light, particularly with some of the generic T4 preparations but also with Synthroid itself which commands about 75% of the market for thyroid preparations. Synthetic T4 preparations have been found to vary in potency from batch to batch. Other batches are not retaining their potency to the expiration date. As a result of these problems in November 1997, the Federal Drug Administration informed the makers of synthetic thyroid preparations, that they had to make new drug applications for their products and will have to prove to the FDA that their products are indeed safe and reliable.[41] They were given a period of about four years to do so. When none met the deadline, it was extended for another year. Currently only one synthetic preparation has received approval---the others are not likely to meet the deadline.

The synthetic T4 products, like the desiccated products, come in many different sizes, varying from 0.012 mg to 0.3 mg. Historically the synthetic products have been regulated by the results from the blood tests. 0.3 mg is usually the maximum dosage

---

[41] **Federal Register;** August, 1997

used.

Various synthetic T3 products are also available. T3 has a half-life in the human body of a little over a day, while T4 has a half-life of around seven days. As a result, T3 preparations have to be taken at least twice a day. Since T3 is more potent than T4, if they do release the stated amount of hormone, one is more apt to see side effects on these pure T3 preparations. Slow release preparations are available through compounding pharmacies, pharmacies which still prepare some of their medications from raw ingredients. In these T3 preparations, the T3 is released over a period of time generally over about twelve hours. It is almost impossible to compound T3 reliably. Many of these slow release preparations have little or no activity. Though the slow release preparations tend to minimize side effects, they are more expensive. Some doctors cycle patients on slow release T3 preparations in an effort to overcome the blockage that exists in T4 to T3 conversion, a problem seen in many individuals. The possible success of this therapy has to be weighed against

THYROID PREPARATIONS

Name	Type of Preparation	Advantages	Disadvantages
Synthroid	Pure T4, Synthetic	blood tests easier to read "consistent" strength	Does not work well (Not converted to T3)
Armour Thyroid	Natural desiccated T3, T4	Many sizes available Patients feel better	
Nature-Throid	Natural desiccated T3, T4	Hypo allergic (no milk or corn) Patients feel better	Not in most pharmacies
Westhroid	Natural desiccated T3, T4	Cheap, Patients feel better	Not in some pharmacies
Cytomel	Synthetic Pure T3	Active hormone	increased side effects
Biotech	Natural desiccated T3, T4	Cheap, Patients feel better	Not in many pharmacies
Slow Release T3	Natural, compounded	Slow release natural hormone	Expensive, increased side effects

hyperthyroid ranges to get results. This therapy often fails due to the generally poor the increased side effects seen since these patients usually have to cycle up into quality of slow-release T3 products. When safer methods of cycling patients are found, this approach may prove more useful. Most clinicians have seen so many problems when this approach has been tried, that they generally do not recommend it.

Some doctors advocate using a blood test for T4 to decide whether or not to use a pure T3 preparation. If the T4 level is low, they will use a desiccated thyroid product. If the T4 is in the high normal range on the blood tests, they will go with a pure T3 preparation. This approach seems to have some merit and should be looked at more closely to see if a better clinical response is obtained.

Adrenal Preparations

When adrenal weakness runs with hypothyroidism, in some ways the dosages are trickier, yet easier at the same time. Most children will do well at a dosage of **prednisone** of about 2.5 mg/day while adults will do well at 5 mg/day or hydrocortisone 2.5 mg four times a day for children and 5 mg four times a day for adults.[42] This dosage should be maintained while thyroid is being increased if they have any signs of adrenal weakness. After the final dosage of thyroid is reached, most of these individuals will be able to come off steroids. The situation is tricky because more options are available, including several over the counter steroid preparations. The human body makes a host of different steroid compounds, closely related in structure but having widely varying biological effects. In fact 150 different steroid compounds produced by the body have been identified which have some biological activity, though these are all grouped into seven main categories, each category with distinct functions. At times these various categories of adrenal hormone need to be balanced out. The categories include, male hormones, female hormones, mineral corticoids (having to do with mineral balance), & glucocorticoids.

Adrenal glandular products are available at most health food stores. Most of these products contain little active hormone, but they contain precursors that the body can use to make active steroids. For this reason they are relatively safe. Even in moderate adrenal insufficiency, however, large amounts may be needed.

DHEA is usually available as well in health food stores. Although it is an adrenal hormone, its actions do not correspond very closely to the glucocorticoids, so it may not meet all the needs in adrenal weakness. It does not play the same role in regulating glucose. Large doses may cause masculinization in women. The biggest

----

[42]William McK. Jeferies MD; **Safe Uses of Cortisone,** 1994

drawback is that when used, acne is often produced, particularly in women. This problem can be minimized by starting on small doses and increasing the dose gradually.[43]

Pregnenolone became available over the counter in the fall of 1996. Many health food stores have not stocked the product since the trade considers all adrenal hormones controversial. Pregnenolone[44] is the first adrenal hormone the body produces from cholesterol and is the precursor for the whole line of steroids the body makes. The rest of the adrenal hormones are manufactured from pregnenolone. If high enough dosages of this hormone are given, one can see any side effect produced by any other steroid depending on how the body utilizes it. It also can correct any type of adrenal deficiency much of the time. Most pregenolone is converted to natural progesterone which can be taken in large amounts without any side effects. So it is relatively safe. It will produce acne in some individuals, even in moderate doses, and others can get fluid retention.

Hydrocortisone is the steroid that is manufactured by the body. When there is no stress, an adult needs 20 mg of hydrocortisone a day. Hydrocortisone has a relatively short half life in the body. In order to keep the body on an even keel, this steroid needs to be taken at least three times a day, preferable four times. When it is taken at night, some individuals have a hard time sleeping. Under stress the body's need for hydrocortisone increases dramatically. Infections, for example, will increase the need for hydrocortisone five fold. So if an individual is taking 20 mg of hydrocortisone, when under stress the dose can be raised to 120 mg. The blood levels do not change, remaining normal in both cases. But once the stress is over, the blood levels will rise on this high dose unless it is decreased. [45] This makes controlling hydrocortisone with blood tests problematical. One must give these hormones based on clinical need. Fortunately the only situation in which this is truly a problem is complete adrenal failure. In most individuals, adding adrenal support merely increases their reserve so their body is able to handle fluctuating needs.

---

[43] Fernard Labra, Alan Belanex et. al.; **Steroids, DHEA & the Intracrine Formation of Androgens & Estrogens;** Vol 6 ,322-328, June 1998.

[44] Fay Sahelian, MD; **Pregnenolone, Nature's Feel Good Hormone,** Avery Publishing Group, 1997.

[45]William McK. Jeferies; **Safe Uses of Cortisone, 1994**

The more often one gives a steroid, the greater the suppression of ones own adrenal glands. Hydrocortisone, which has to be given three times a day actually causes four to fives times more suppression than does prednisone, which can be given once a day. In cliniccal studies five to 7.5 mg of prednisone did not cause any suppression of one's own adrenals. So this dosage range is extremely safe. It takes dosages of prednisone in excess of 15 mg a day to cause complete suppression of the adrenal. [46] Most individuals on prolonged prednisone therapy a dosage of even 15 mg or less can undergo major stress without any additional adrenal support.

With so many steroid preparations available which have such differing effects, it is not surprising that more than one preparation may need to be given. Not only do adrenal hormones have to be balanced with thyroid, they may have to be balanced with one another. Much more clinical experience is needed in this area. For example, estrogen at the present time is often given in dosages that upset the balance of other

Adrenal Preparations:

Name	Preparation	Advantages	Disadvantages
Adrenal Glandular	Desiccated gland	Few side effects, Strengthens own gland	Inconsistent, not very potent
Pregnenolone	Adrenal hormone---Precursor	Safe---Precursor of all other adrenal hormones	Difficult to find -Not carried by many
DHEA	Adrenal hormone	Safe, available Balances glucocorticoids	Not a glucocorticoid Masculinization
Prednisone	Synthetic glucocorticoid	Single day dose Cheap	Not as effective in some individuals
Hydrocortisone	Natural glucocorticoid	Same as body makes	Must take 4x day More side effects

hormones. Better results for overall health will often result with smaller doses of estrogen, and the side effect profile may be greatly reduced including that of increased cancer .

When thyroid and steroids are used together, their side effects are minimized.

---

[46]Harry E. Klinefelter MD et. al.; **Single Daily Dose Predisone,** JAMA, Vol 241 pp 2721-2723, 1979.

Dr. Barnes, for example, had 1,500 patients on a combination of thyroid and prednisone. He never saw a significant side effect on this regimen. **The secret is in giving medications within physiologic dosages ranges, doses which are no greater than a normal individual should produce. When this is done, both thyroid and steroids are among the safest medications available**. Used in this fashion, they are able to live up to their early reputation as miracle drugs.

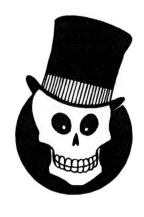

Chapter 9   **Complications of Therapy**

Tony was given less than six months to live. He had repeated strokes. Surgery on his carotids had not corrected the problem. He was told he could expect another major stroke at any time. He also had symptoms of hypothyroidism. He was cold and tired. He was irritable. His skin was dry. And he had a low basal temperature. He was started on a half grain of thyroid and gradually the dosage was increased to 3 grains. of thyroid. He never did have another stroke. He had nearly six good years and then began developing angina. His thyroid dosage was cut down, but the angina persisted. Two years later a cardiologist who was consulted decided to try bypass surgery. He died two weeks later of surgical complications.

Tony although very ill, had his life prolonged by taking thyroid hormones. Thyroid, when it is used properly, is one of the safest medications available. On the basis of pure theory, if one were to start at a small dose of thyroid and increase that dosage gradually, thyroid should be virtually without side effects, even if the dosage needed was exceeded. One should not get side effects until the physiologic dose is exceeded. The feedback mechanisms which have already been discussed will keep the blood levels of thyroid unchanged as long as the increase in dosage is truly gradual. In a normal individual one should not be able to give enough thyroid to appreciably change thyroid function until a dosage of four and one half grains is exceeded in a small individual, or five grains in a larger individual---toward the upper limit of the physiologic dosage range. Above this dosage one may start seeing hyperthyroid symptoms. In a few individuals, poor absorption or antibodies to thyroid hormone result in larger doses being needed and individuals will remain euthyroid on doses of 8 grs or more.

In practice one can and often will see side effects at smaller dosages of thyroid hormone. The more severe the hypothyroidism, the more likely problems are to arise when replacement therapy is started. For some reason being low thyroid leaves an individual supersensitive to the effects of thyroid hormone. Though in most individuals a starting dose of 1 gr of desiccated thyroid is very well tolerated and even starting dosages of 2 grs are without unwanted side effects in most young men, these dosages are not tolerated in some who are severely hypothyroid. Even when adrenal support is added these individuals cannot tolerate a 1 gr dosage. They feel jittery and develop other symptoms like palpitations which are produced by an excess of thyroid hormone.

The starting dosage will have to be dropped in these individuals. No neat formula exists to tell what the initial dosage should be for these patients. In some supersensitive individuals, one may need to start at a dosage as low as 1/16th of a grain, much smaller than the initial dosage for an infant. It will take time and patience to finally bring them up to a dosage of thyroid hormone that will get rid of their hypothyroid symptoms---in some cases two years or more. Clinical experience says about five percent of patients will fall into the sensitive category and most of these will do well at a starting dose of ½ gr. But one must be prepared for the supersensitive patient.

There is a second group of patients in which starting on a smaller dose, generally ½ grain of desiccated thyroid, is imperative. These are the individuals with underlying heart problems. Since thyroid increases metabolism, which means the amount of energy expended by the body will be increased, any extra thyroid will increase the work load on the heart. If the vessels going to the heart are partially blocked by plaques from arteriosclerosis, an oxygen debt to the heart may occur due to the decreased blood supply available. This may bring on angina, which is heart or cardiac pain. Large initial doses of thyroid hormone or a large increase in dosage given under these circumstances can prove fatal. On the other hand, if the dosage is increased slowly, by 1/4 gr increments, the individual can eventually be increased without any problem to a dosage of 2 grs. of thyroid, the recommended dose for people with severe heart problems.[47]

By far the most common side effects from taking thyroid are due to its inter-relationship with the adrenal and its hormones. This subject is covered in detail in the chapter discussing this relationship. In brief, taking thyroid speeds up the metabolism of adrenal hormone. This may leave inadequate adrenal hormones to meet the needs of the body. All the symptoms associated with hypothyroidism may worsen. In addition the pulse may speed up, allergies may worsen and the individual may develop such things as panic attacks or palpitations. Adding adrenal support will get rid of most of these symptoms. In fact a trial of adrenal support is warranted if the patient feels worse in any way when placed on thyroid. Another tactic available and used by some is to increase the thyroid much more gradually than usual---in the same increments as with heart patients, 1/4 gr at a time with an interval of up to two months between dosage increases. This tactic will avoid most of these side effects. But it will take much longer to reach the dosage level that will get rid of their hypothyroid

---

[47]Broda O. Barnes, Charlotte W. Barnes; **Solved: The Riddle of Heart Attacks**, Robinson Press, 1978.

symptoms. For the average adult this is about 3 grs of thyroid. Most individuals will not need to change the dosage once the correct dosage has been determined but will be maintained at the same dosage for years.

One must also be aware of the effects that an increased metabolism has on other functions of the body. The increased metabolism can result in a number of deficiencies if no attention is given to vitamin and mineral replacement. Perhaps the earliest deficiency to be documented was a deficiency of some of the B vitamins such as B6 which occurred in patients on thyroid replacement therapy   Without a supplemental B vitamin intake this is a common occurrence..[48]   More recently B12 deficiency has been found to be a problem. Hypothyroid patients lack stomach acid. This can translate into a B12 deficiency for an intrinsic factor is not available which is essential for the absorption of Vitamin B12. Again, increasing the metabolism increases the need for all these vitamins.

One of the chief concerns which is currently expressed by the medical profession is the danger of excess thyroid causing osteoporosis. The initial concern was raised from the data on hyperthyroidism, which indeed is associated with an increase in osteoporosis in research studies. The evidence has not been as clear cut when what is felt to be an excess dosage of thyroid is given to treat hypothyroidism. This evidence is based on TSH testing, on low TSH levels where the TSH seems to be suppressed. The conclusion which is reached is that the individual must be on too much thyroid, though this conclusion is usually incorrect. For in these individuals, there is no clinical evidence of hyperthyroidism and temperatures are normal. The problem with most of these studies is that calcium intake was not considered, not even mentioned in the studies. *There are studies in which individuals were given too much thyroid based on their TSH results, but also given excellent calcium supplementation and were found to have no problem as far as their bones were concerned.* They did not develop osteoporosis. The research on osteoporosis is confounded by the fact that hypothyroid patients have thick, but weak bones. These bones thin out but become stronger on thyroid replacement therapy. Research will likely eventually show that any increased osteoporosis with supposed excess thyroid intake is due to a relative calcium and magnesium deficiency produced by the increased metabolism seen when thyroid levels are restored to normal. Most of the studies have been done on the synthetic thyroid hormones which do not completely normalize thyroid function so are suspect for that

---

[48]Broda O. Barnes, Lawrence Galton; **Hypothyroidism: The Unsuspected Illness**, Thomas Y. Crowell Company, 1976.

reason alone. Marathon runners develop osteoporosis for much the same reason as seen in these studies---higher metabolic activity with no increase in calcium intake.

The theory *that extra thyroid will cause osteoporosis* seems absurd in light of the fact that thyroid levels are much higher in young children than in adults. The greatest growth in the skeleton takes place in the first year of life when the weight of a child triples. The thyroid levels at this time are actually ten times higher than levels found in an adult. It is hard to see that a small amount of extra thyroid could cause too many problems for the skeleton in light of this fact---massive growth of the skeleton occurs when thyroid levels are elevated in childhood. Some doctors believe that thyroid may actually help prevent osteoporosis and strengthen the bones, but more research is needed.

Some doctors are concerned with the palpitations which can occur when thyroid is given. Yesterday's literature stated that when palpitations occurred, they almost always went away with time if the same dosage was maintained. This leads to the belief that palpitations are basically a symptom of imbalance of thyroid and adrenal functions since low adrenal function which co-exists with hypothyroidism improves over time in most hypothyroid patients who are placed on thyroid therapy. It may be that the palpitations associated with hyperthyroidism are due to a relative adrenal insufficiency and might be improved greatly with adrenal hormones. A clinical study of this point would be informative.

Other deficiencies may occur when thyroid is started, but at this time they are not as well documented. But paying attention to overall nutrition is important for the hypothyroid patient in light of the increased metabolism seen in replacement therapy.

The food one eats does have a role to play in thyroid therapy. It is well known that certain foods, particularly members of the cabbage family if eaten raw in large amounts, will suppress thyroid function, for they contain anti-thyroid substances. This is rarely a problem with the American diet. A growing problem is the amount of soy protein ingested particularly among vegetarians. The estrogen like effects of soy protein suppress thyroid function and can cause goiter.

Other foods can decrease the absorption of thyroid. Many, therefore, recommend that thyroid be taken on an empty stomach. Iron supplements likely have the greatest clinical importance, though other minerals like calcium may suppress absorption to a much lesser extent. Iron interferes greatly enough with the absorption of thyroid, so the two should not be taken together. This includes vitamins that have large iron contents.

Foods have other effects as well. A high protein diet increases the need for thyroid. If one changes from a high protein to a high carbohydrate diet, the need for thyroid will decrease. On the other hand, lack of protein or the consumption of only poor quality proteins will also slow thyroid function. Some of these relationships must be kept in mind, and if need for thyroid seems to change inquiries as to dietary changes should be made.

Thyroid hormone is a very potent medication, so the tablets have inert ingredients that make up most of the their bulk. Individuals can be sensitive to these inert ingredients even though the amounts are small enough that this is rarely a problem. Absorption can be affected by these ingredients, and at times it is helpful to change preparation if one does not observe the desired response on what should be an adequate dose of thyroid.

In general, the side effects one will see while taking physiologic doses of thyroid are minor and are easily controlled. They should not prevent anyone from receiving adequate thyroid therapy.

Tina developed lupus many years ago. Though her disease didn't progress, the treatment of her lupus did not get rid of many of her symptoms. She was tired, lacked the energy to keep up with a regular work schedule. Thyroid replacement therapy got rid of these nagging symptoms. Of equal importance, the thyroid seemed to stabilize the lupus. Her big problem had been with her platelets. These would drop to dangerous levels, levels which would prevent her blood from clotting. Thus, she could bleed uncontrollably with any slight injury if she was not treated with large doses of steroids, doses which were producing many side effects. By taking the thyroid, she has been well maintained for years on small physiologic doses of steroid, doses which have produced no side effects. She feels much better in other ways as well. Her crippling tiredness is a thing of the past and she has been able to lead a productive life. She has now reached retirement age but is still going strong.

Thyroid hormone may help individuals like Tina for it has been discovered that the cells of the body communicate with each other. They do so through a 'language" that is printed on the surface of the individual cells. This 'language' is made up of an alphabet consisting of eight different simple sugars. Though some of these sugars can be manufactured by the body, it is advantageous to have even these provided in the diet, for it is difficult for the body to manufacture sufficient quantities of the sugars it uses in this communication scheme. Only a few of these sugars are present in any significant amount in the diets of the average American today, and they are usually not present in adequate quantities. These sugars are capable of being twisted into many different stable shapes or configurations. In fact, just four of these different sugars taken together can form more than 100,000 different patterns or "words." Just what information the cells communicate to each other is not known. But the amount of information communicated could be almost unlimited. This is one of the hot areas of research today. The information exchanged is sufficient so that the cells work together in harmony to carry out the special purposes of each organ, or collection of cells. Such information as the type of cells that each individual cell is supposed to be joined to on each of its sides and where blood vessels should run is information that would need to be included; thus information on how the cells are to be organized into a functioning organ is spelled out. If the body is not able to produce sufficient amounts of the needed sugars, if the words printed on the surface of the cells are no longer correct, or complete, the ability of the cells to communicate with each other breaks down. Recent research shows that this breakdown in communication between cells is occurring in the autoimmune diseases studied. The sugar words are being misprinted on the surface of the cells so the cells can no longer exchange the information necessary for them to function as a cohesive unit.[49]

Certainly it is critical to get sufficient amounts of these sugars in the diet, but there are other factors leading to the breakdown of this cellular communication system as well. One autoimmune disease that has been extensively studied is rheumatoid arthritis, a disease that often develops in young adults and sometimes will severely cripple them. Some researchers postulate that at least three factors enter into the development of rheumatoid arthritis. Two of these relate to the adrenal gland. In order to develop rheumatoid arthritis researchers believe the individual must be low in both glucocorticoids and in DHEA.[50] They then believe a low grade infection is present in the joints, frequently caused by a chlamydia type organism that acts as the trigger to initiate the whole autoimmune process. When the resistance of the body is down due to low adrenal function, this infectious agent initiates the partial or complete destruction of the sugar layer of the cell membrane, thus resulting in a loss of communication between the cells. The loss of communication results in further destruction of tissue. In the case of rheumatoid arthritis, the cartilage in joints is eventually destroyed as the cartilage cells are no longer recognized by other cells as legitimate parts of the body. The ultimate result is full blown rheumatoid arthritis.

In an autoimmune illness when the body is no longer able to recognize the cells that are stripped of their proper identification markers, it develops antibodies to them. This will result in the destruction of the cells involved, as described in rheumatoid arthritis, where the body develops antibodies against joint tissue. But when the body still recognizes the cells as belonging (as a part of the body) although they may not be functioning normally, auto-antibodies are not produced and can not be measured in the blood stream in abnormal quantities though the individual has symptoms of disease. This fact indicates that it is the loss of communication between the cells that is the primary problem underlying autoimmune disease. If a cell has lost most of the identifying code words on its surface, if it can no longer tell other cells it is a member of a properly functioning organ, the body treats it as an unwanted invader rather than a vital part of the cellular community. In other words, the body starts producing

---

[49] **Mannatec Products;** Information sheets

[50] William McK Jefferies MD; **Mild Adrenocortical Deficiency, Chronic allergies**; Medical Hypotheses, Vol 42, pp 183-189, 1994.

antibodies against these cells to get rid of them as not belonging and as potentially dangerous. So if the disease process is mild, if communication between cells, although disrupted, has not completely broken down and the body is still able to recognize that the cells involved are a proper part of the body, actual tissue destruction should not occur. It is when cells are no longer recognized as a proper part of the body that auto-antibodies arise and the body actually turns on itself in a major destructive way.

Various members of the adrenal system are involved in this process. Women tend to suffer more from autoimmune disease than men do. Estrogen enhances the vigilance of the body against any foreign invasion, enhances the ability of the body to recognize cells as abnormal or foreign. *Progesterone on the other hand relaxes this vigilance*. If women have excessive levels of estrogen, they are more likely to develop autoimmune problems. The high levels of estrogen seen in pregnancy are thus likely responsible for the autoimmune antibodies to thyroid seen in women following childbirth.

What does this autoimmune process have to do with thyroid function? First let's review some very general relationships. Hypothyroidism slows down the functioning of the adrenal gland. This alone helps set the stage for the development of autoimmune disease. Hypothyroidism also decreases the resistance to infections which are known to play a part in several autoimmune diseases. When an individual is low thyroid, when the metabolism is sluggish, many body processes are not functioning at full capacity, many enzyme systems are hampered. Generalized sluggishness ensues, which results in a greater susceptibility to chronic disease. But there is a specific relationship of thyroid to autoimmune disease. To understand this relationship a discussion of myxedema is important.

Myxedema refers to mucous compounds which collect in the body when individuals are severely hypothyroid, and severe hypothyroidism is often simply called myxedema. Mucous compounds are made up of polysaccharides, complex compounds made up of many different sugar units. Certain kinds of mucous polysaccharides play an important role in individuals who have hypothyroidism. When the hypothyroidism is severe these mucous like compounds become a prominent feature of the disease. These polysaccharides build up in large quantities in the tissues of the body as a result of inadequate thyroid function. The very presence of these polysaccharides causes some of the symptoms and physical findings in hypothyroidism. For example, these complex sugars bind strongly to water, producing excess water retention that can result in swelling of the hands and feet in hypothyroid patients. Early researchers were amazed when they did autopsies on individuals who died with severe myxedema, because although their bodies were bloated due to excess water content, the tissues actually appeared dry since these polysaccharides held onto the excess water so tightly. Almost no seepage of serous fluid would take place where these bodies were cut open. In the average individual with even mild thyroid deficiency, the body retains about six extra pounds of water, held onto by these complex sugars. This excess water weight will be lost as the body gets rid of these polysaccharides when thyroid therapy is started. [51]

These complex sugars, the myxedema of hypothyroidism, are similar to the sugars which are involved in the communication between cells. It is possible that these polysaccharides are a result of either a defect in the manufacture of the communicating sugar layer of the cells or an inability to get rid of the complex sugars lining the surface of the cells when these cells are replaced due to normal wear and tear. In any case the presence of these polysaccharides in hypothyroidism is bound to interfere with the communication between the cells. Sugar fragments floating between the cells will act as noise jamming the communication. The normal cells are confused by reading free floating sugar messages which have no relevance to the actual messages nearby cells are trying to give. Further, the polysaccarides can act as a barrier between cells just by taking up space, making the cells communicate with each other through a greater distance. Getting rid of this extra noise is crucial for cells to be able to communicate efficiently, and it may become critical if cells have already sustained significant damage through an autoimmune process.

Treating individuals with autoimmune diseases with thyroid therefore is important for it will help reestablish the proper communication between cells. This allows patients who traditionally have been treated with high doses of steroids to be treated with steroid doses that are physiologic, doses that are no greater than the body normally puts out. Low, physiologic dose therapy avoids all the horrible side effects which are produced by large doses of steroids. Clinical experience in a limited number of individuals with autoimmune diseases indicates that their symptoms are usually well controlled with physiologic doses of both thyroid and steroids. In the light of the fact that different steroids are important in the development of autoimmune problems, more

---

[51] L. Ross McDougall; **Thyroid Disease in Clinical Practice**, Oxford University Press, 1992.

attention needs to be given to balancing the various steroid components in these conditions as well.

These complex sugars may impact thyroid function in another fashion. It is interesting that TSH, thyroid stimulating hormone, itself, has complex sugars in its make up. Again, if some of these sugars are not available in adequate amounts, the TSH that the body produces may be defective. Hormone levels may look normal in the tests being run for TSH, but lack of the proper sugars in TSH's structure can destroy its activity and so it will not release an adequate amount of thyroid hormone, T4, from the thyroid gland even when the gland has adequate hormonal stores. These individuals with an abnormal TSH are functionally hypothyroid, having a type of secondary hypothyroidism.[52] When the body is having problems with its sugar coding in autoimmune disease, it is probable that sugar problems are present in other areas of the body, such as with the sugar in TSH. In any case, in a number of autoimmune diseases it is known that subtle problems occur in the pituitary- hypothalamus axis because some elements of secondary hypothyroidism are present.

Much of the information in this chapter is on the cutting edge of research. Much more research needs to be done. Perhaps if the contribution of hypothyroidism to autoimmune problems is fully understood, significant progress will be made in controlling these devastating diseases.

---

[52]Lewis E. Braverman; **Werner & Ingbar's The Thyroid,** Lippincott & Ravens Publishers, 1996.

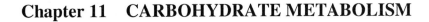

Chapter 11   CARBOHYDRATE METABOLISM

In the mid-eighties Sherry developed symptoms that at first were minor but gradually increased in severity. Though tired all the time she was not able to get a good night's rest and her weight was gradually creeping up. She was constantly cold and complained of hypoglycemic symptoms. She was told by physicians whom she consulted that her symptoms were consistent with hypothyroidism. *But since all her blood tests came back in the low normal range, nothing was done about it.* Her temperature and blood pressure were so low that often in the doctor's office the nurse would double check them to make sure they were correct. The hypoglycemic attacks became worse; she often became dizzy, hot, and clammy. Her tongue felt thickened. At times she would have to sit down for fear of falling or passing out. In the spring of 1996 she was finally placed on natural desiccated thyroid. Soon all her symptoms were gone and she felt well. Her hypoglycemic attacks were just a memory. Life had become worth living for her again.

As Sherry discovered correcting hypothyroidism is a key to controlling hypoglycemia. We already explained that thyroid hormones control the burning of the main fuel of the body, glucose, while the adrenal hormones, the glucocorticoids, control its release from various storage depots. One would expect significant problems in sugar metabolism if either of these hormones is lacking and this is indeed the case. They are important both in hypoglycemia where the sugar levels in the blood drop too low and in diabetes where the sugar levels are too high. But there are other actors in these dramas that one needs to know about, actors that can help control some of the symptoms of hypothyroidism by helping to see that normal carbohydrate metabolism takes place in the body.

The first of these actors are the minerals. Minerals are important for enzymes to work properly and often appear as co-factors that enhance the speed of chemical reactions. Often a half dozen or more different minerals are involved in a single reaction, most of the time necessary in only trace amounts. Some of these minerals may be key players in a given reaction, while others may merely increase the efficiency of the chemical reactions a bit. Though mineral deficiencies are common, some occur much more frequently than others. Some minerals like zinc and magnesium are involved in so many different chemical reactions in the body that they are needed in fairly large quantities. [53] Their role in sugar metabolism is almost taken for granted.

Selenium may play a role in carbohydrate metabolism simply because selenium is an essential part of both type 1 and type 3 de-iodinase, [54] and thus supports thyroid function. De-iodinases, as discussed in the chapter on thyroid metabolism, regulate the formation of T3 and RT3. T3, the most active thyroid hormone, enhances the entry of sugar into the cells. If not enough selenium is present, the cells may not receive enough carbohydrate to burn. However, the body guards the selenium in these enzymes (the de-iodinases) and so they are the last to be depleted of their selenium when there is not enough to go around. Therefore, other selenium containing enzymes are impacted first, causing profound effects in the areas where they should be active, particularly in the immune system. These effects are usually so severe that any mild effect on sugar metabolism is hidden.

Two trace minerals stand out as important actors in sugar metabolism. The first is **vanadium**. Like insulin, vanadium enhances the entry of glucose into cells from the bloodstream and to a certain extent can replace the need for insulin. Just how it works is not understood. **Chromium** is the other important mineral. Certain chromium-containing molecules are involved in the delivery to and utilization of fat by the mitochondria---the chemical factories of the cells. In other words chromium is necessary for the body to tap into its main energy reservoir, fat.

When chromium and vanadium are lacking in the diet, which unfortunately is true for most Americans today, these individuals will develop insulin resistance over a period of time. In insulin resistance, it takes more insulin than usual to process the same amount of glucose, so the body has to produce more insulin to meet the ordinary needs of metabolism. With the tremendous increase in refined carbohydrates in the American diet, coupled with key mineral deficiencies, it is no wonder that over half the population shows signs of insulin resistance. A century ago the average individual in this country ate five to ten pounds of refined carbohydrate such as table sugar in a year's time. Today most Americans eat that much in a week. This tremendous increase in the sugar load has placed more demands on carbohydrate metabolism than

---

[53]Joel D. Wallach, BS, DVM, ND, Ma Lan, MD, MS; **Rare Earths---Forbidden Cures**; Double Happiness Publishing Company, May 1995.

[54] Sing-yung Wu, Theo L. Vissar et. al.; **Thyroid Hormone Metabolism-Molecular Biology**; CRC Press, 1994.

many individuals can adequately handle.   But to gain further insight into   the carbohydrate story the role of   three actors in the carbohydrate drama must be discussed.   The first of these is insulin.

The best-known property of **insulin** is its ability to control the entry of glucose into the cells.   When not enough insulin is produced, sugar levels rise in the blood because the glucose is not entering into the cells in a proper fashion. Insulin's other important task is that of a storage hormone. It not only puts glucose into cells so the body can obtain energy through burning this sugar fuel, it also places any extra glucose, actually any extra calories, into fat storage. In fact, when insulin levels are high, it prevents fat from being used by the body. So insulin increases the rate in which fuel is being burned by helping it enter the cells and blocks the procurement of additional fuel from fat at the same time. So another hormone is needed to balance this situation out. That hormone is glucagon.

Glucagon enhances and regulates the release of glucose from its storage deposits. If blood sugar levels are low, glucagon, when present in sufficient amounts, will bring the levels up almost immediately. So glucagon is a useful medication in hypoglycemic attacks where blood levels of sugar drop too low. It also helps mobilize the fat stores of the body, helping fat enter the mitochondria to be burned.

One other effect of insulin should be mentioned. The cells of the body have powerful hormones called ecchinoids or prostaglandins that help control the cell's functions. These are manufactured from the essential fatty acids consumed in the diet. For instance, some of these prostaglandins will raise blood pressure, others will lower it. Some prostaglandins increase inflammation in body tissues, others decrease this same inflammation. Insulin has a regulating effect on these prostaglandins, tending to increase the prostaglandins which produce unwanted side effects such as inflammation when insulin levels are high. So to maintain good health it is important to keep the levels of insulin low and on an even keel.

The third actor in the story are the fats and oils in the diet or rather the trans fatty acids that are formed when fats and oils are heated.   The polyunsaturated oils that make up so much of the current American diet are the real culprits, for they are unstable and change structure when heated. Fatty acids make up an important portion of the membranes of all cells. When trans fatty acids, fatty acids that have an abnormal three dimensional structure, become incorporated into the cellular membranes, it becomes difficult for insulin to move glucose into the cells normally. In the average American diet, 20 to 30% of the fat calories are from trans fatty acids. Contrary to popular belief, saturated fats are not detrimental to health. Margarine and other man made saturated fats have been lumped in with animal fat in research data bases. These man made fats are even higher in trans fatty acids, approaching levels of 50%, than are the polyunsaturated oils. It is these fats that are causing the problems such as heart disease that the saturated fats have been blamed for. The improper fats in our diets have had a major impact on carbohydrate metabolism in this country and are starting to be recognized as a major player in insulin resistance.

Insulin is produced by the body in response to carbohydrate or sugar intake. A high carbohydrate diet demands higher insulin levels. High insulin levels put all extra calories into fat. What is worse, this fat cannot be utilized but merely sits in storage. Individuals get hungry sooner than they should, for they cannot touch their main energy reserves, fat. Instead they have to eat to maintain their blood sugar. Glucagon, on the other hand, is controlled by the protein intake in the diet. An adequate protein intake is needed to provide a sufficient quantity of glucagon to allow the body to tap its fat reserves for energy. [55]

A balance between carbohydrate and protein consumption is critical if the body is to function in a normal, efficient fashion. Actually both the minerals, chromium and vanadium, and the metabolic regulating hormones, the thyroid and glucocorticoids, are important in this picture. If these minerals or hormones are lacking, the balance between carbohydrate and protein intake becomes much more critical. A balanced intake of calories occurs when one gets about 40% carbohydrate, 30% protein and 30% fat in the diet. If the glucocorticoid and thyroid levels were ideal, an individual might have no problems on a diet of 70% carbohydrate, 15% protein and 15% fat. But most Americans on this kind of carbohydrate-heavy diet would have to eat starvation rations in order to lose weight and would not feel good trying to do so. When carbohydrate and protein calories are balanced, an overweight person can often eat normal amounts of food and still lose weight.

We are now ready to discuss problems in sugar metabolism as they relate to hypothyroidism. The first of these is hypoglycemia which is much more common than diabetes. The primary defect in hypoglycemia is a relative lack of the glucocorticoids and a corresponding inability to release sufficient glucose from storage depots in the body. When blood sugar levels are low, individuals start feeling light-headed, weak

---

[55] Barry Sears; **Enter The Zone**, 1995.

and sweaty. The brain depends on glucose alone for its metabolic needs. The rest of the body has back up systems which can break down fat or protein for fuel that can be put into play if needed for energy production, so the glucose levels are not as crucial for other areas of the body. If glucose levels are low enough, an individual can quickly slip into unconsciousness. One rule in medicine is that all individuals who are comatose should be treated as if they have low blood sugar if the cause of the coma is not known. Prolonged hypoglycemia will damage brain cells killing some of them.

The production and release of adrenalin is part of a back up system which is activated when blood sugar levels are low. Adrenalin releases sugar stores and brings up glucose levels in the bloodstream. In hypothyroidism much more adrenalin is released than in normal individuals as the body seeks to maintain its sugar levels. In fact some hypothyroid individuals will actually release thirty times the normal amounts of adrenalin for this purpose.

Often when the body attempts to respond to the low blood sugar, it produces too much insulin. There is a mismatch between what the body produces and what is needed to process the carbohydrates in the diet. The presence of excess insulin will produce symptoms. We mentioned insulin can increase inflammation, so aches and pains often increase when individuals have problems with hypoglycemia. Frontal headaches are common when blood sugar levels are low. When individuals have a tendency toward hypoglycemia, it is common for the sugar levels in the blood to drop in the middle of the night. This is more likely to occur if a carbohydrate bedtime snack has been consumed. When blood sugar levels drop these individuals will wake up and have a hard time going back to sleep while the blood sugar levels remain low. The low sugar levels disturb the functioning of the brain just enough to make sleep difficult. The reason is not known. These individuals may not be able to get back to sleep unless they eat a snack. So hypoglycemia contributes to insomnia.

A further problem is that insulin has a profound effect on the intercellular environment--- for example it changes the potassium levels in the cells. This in turn affects their functioning. The greatest effects are seen in the central nervous system. Individuals often will feel nervous and irritated as a result of the altered intercellular environment. Temper outbursts occur commonly, at times for trivial reasons, and clarity of thinking often becomes clouded.

The effect of alcohol on hypoglycemia should be mentioned for this reaction is worse in hypothyroidism. Alcohol blocks the release of glucose from the liver's glycogen stores. In young children this blockage is long lasting and profound. In a young child, alcohol can produce such a severe hypoglycemia that it can actually kill the child. Alcohol causes hypoglycemia in adults as well, but this hypoglycemia tends to be much milder. Heredity plays a significant role in how severe this problem will be. An important mechanism behind intoxication with alcohol is the lowering of blood glucose levels to the point the brain is no longer able to function properly. So when an individual is drunk, it is the lack of glucose in the brain that is causing his behavior, rather than a toxic effect of alcohol. These sugar levels often become low enough so that brain cells are killed; at least a few brain cells are destroyed each time an individual becomes drunk. [56]

Hypoglycemia means cells everywhere in the body are not getting sufficient fuel. This lack of glucose in turn shuts down the conversion of T4 to T3. Hypoglycemia itself produces a functional hypothyroidism and thus will produce all the other symptoms of hypothyroidism.   Once initiated, hypoglycemia can lead to a vicious cycle with ever worsening symptoms unless carbohydrate intake is controlled. Foods should be chosen that have a low glycemic index, in other words foods that will not raise the blood sugar to any great extent.

The situation with diabetes is more complex. Juvenile diabetes is an autoimmune disorder which indicates adrenal weakness. Adrenal weakness now appears to be a part of all autoimmune disorders. A viral trigger seems to be responsible for initiating the process of destruction in the pancreas of the beta cells which produce insulin for the body. In addition, at least twenty percent of juvenile diabetics have antibodies to thyroid and eventually ten percent of these juvenile type diabetics will develop primary hypothyroidism. Eventually enough thyroid tissue is destroyed so that it is unable to release adequate quantities of thyroid.

In adult onset diabetics, insulin resistance occurs and insulin levels are high at the onset of the problem.   As mentioned, this is a result of the excess carbohydrate intake of most Americans.   Lack of essential minerals contributes to this problem. Unfortunately excess weight (and Americans are becoming fatter) adds to this problem. Excess weight increases insulin resistance by decreasing the number of insulin binding sites that are available. Just losing weight will often restore sugar metabolism to normal. There is also a mismatch between insulin production and the

---

[56] Broda O Barnes MD, Charlotte W. Barnes; **Hope for Hypoglycemia**; Robinson Press, 1978.

requirements of the body in adult onset diabetics, so mild hypoglycemic events are also common. Eventually the pancreas becomes exhausted and is no longer able to put out sufficient quantities of insulin, thus insulin shots may be needed in adult onset diabetics.

In diabetes, since glucose has a difficult time entering cells, the cells of the body are starved for fuel. How this difficulty is aggravated by the incorporation of trans fatty acids into the lipid layers which distorts the cellular membranes making the passage of glucose into the cells has been described. The resulting lack of fuel will automatically shut down the production of T3 from T4 in the cells, causing virtually all diabetics to become functionally hypothyroid. Many of the worst complications of diabetes are markedly aggravated by this underlying hypothyroidism, particularly the vascular complications and some of the neurologic complications of the disease. But those types of problems are subjects of other chapters.

The high sugar levels in the blood become breeding grounds for bacterial and fungal invaders, and the resistance of the body is not great enough to fight these invaders off. Again, in the fact that these infections are generally severe, the effects of diabetes are being aggravated by the underlying hypothyroidism. Individuals who are hypothyroid tend to be dehydrated; they just do not drink normal amounts of water. High sugar levels in the blood, when high enough, act as a diuretic pulling water out of the body through the kidneys. This increases the dehydration and is severe enough at times in diabetics to constitute a medical emergency. The dehydration of diabetes may be aggravated by the underlying hypothyroid connection.

The treatment of this underlying hypothyroidism is critical if diabetic individuals are to function in a normal fashion. Unless the underlying hypothyroidism is corrected, diabetics can look forward to major medical problems. It has been estimated that the lifetime cost of diabetes is in the $300,000 to $400,000 dollar range. And who can put a price on good health? Poor health is not a price diabetics need to pay. An understanding of the relationship of diabetes to hypothyroidism is critical. The hypothyroidism needs to be corrected to prevent many of the complications of diabetes. But until this relationship is understood, diabetes will continue to be the curse it has been.

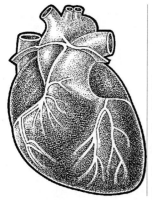

Chapter 12   The Circulatory System

Susan was a brittle diabetic who had struggled to maintain her sugar levels for nearly ten years when she was first seen for hypothyroid symptoms. Her sugar levels frequently ran very high and she constantly had to change her insulin dosage to try to keep those sugar levels under control. But what was worse, she was starting to develop vascular complications. Her ophthalmologist told her that likely within two months she would need surgery on the micro-aneurysms that were developing in her eyes. She had the tiredness, the low basal temperature and other symptoms that went with a low thyroid condition---symptoms shared by most diabetics; most of them are hypothyroid due to their faulty carbohydrate metabolism. She was started on thyroid and her dosage was gradually increased to three grains of thyroid a day. She still had to struggle to maintain her blood sugar at a proper level, though even this became somewhat easier for her as her brittle diabetes stabilized. Her tiredness and other symptoms improved. After eight years, a job change meant she and her husband moved so her subsequent history is not known. But for those eight years she went to her ophthalmologist several times a year. He would shake his head each time and say, "Your eyes have not changed, have not gotten any worse. In fact they seem somewhat better. You don't need any laser surgery yet." Therapy with thyroid had stopped the progression of her vascular problems.

Perhaps the biggest single impact that correcting hypothyroidism may have is on the cardiovascular disease. Susan greatly benefitted from this therapy. Other than cancer, no problem medicine faces causes as much grief as does the ravages of arteriosclerosis. Not only does it underlie the majority of deaths that take place in our society, but relatively young men and less frequently women are snatched away in the midst of their productive years. For other individuals it means living with paralysis for years following a stroke, which suddenly makes it almost impossible to cope with the simple chores of everyday living. For a few it means a descent into dementia where the mind is destroyed and total dependence on a care-giver becomes essential.

Dr. Broda Barnes wrote a small book called, **Solved, the Riddle of Heart Attacks,**.[57] in which he told of his clinical experience with the prevention of heart

---

[57]Broda O Barnes MD, Charlotte Barnes; **Solved the Riddle of Heart Attacks**; Robinson press; 1976.

disease in using desiccated thyroid The impact of thyroid on vascular disease has not been appreciated, largely due to the fact that synthetic T4 preparations of thyroid have been the drugs of choice in thyroid disease for the last thirty years, and these preparations do not have nearly the impact on hardening of the arteries, at least not in the doses used, as do the natural desiccated products. For example, studies done on individuals who were classified as having subclinical hypothyroidism---individuals who had TSH levels above normal but whose levels had not risen into a definite hypothyroid range and had little if any clinical symptoms---have been given Synthroid in an effort to lower their cholesterol. [58] (The relationship between an elevated cholesterol and hypothyroidism has long been known. An elevated cholesterol level was even proposed as a laboratory test for hypothyroidism at one time.) The results of the thyroid therapy in these individuals were disappointing. The most dramatic finding, the results of a single research group, was a lowering of the cholesterol in a group of these individuals by twenty percent. But other research groups found no difference at all between those taking Synthroid and those taking a placebo.

Contrast this with the experience of Dr. Barnes in using natural desiccated thyroid. He did a study in which every single individual who came into his office with a cholesterol above 220, some with levels above 300, was placed on thyroid. After he had more than one thousand patients in the study, he followed them for a minimum of two years. Only one individual dropped out of the study after developing palpitations. Dr. Barnes was able to bring the cholesterol down to normal levels in 99% of these individuals by appropriately increasing their thyroid dose. Most of them were well controlled with a dose no greater than 3 grs. of thyroid, and all were controlled with physiologic doses of thyroid---the dosage that their own glands should be putting out if they had normal thyroid function. He then matched these patients in his study with the ongoing Framingham study, a study in New England on the development of disease in an average American community.   During the time period in which Dr. Barnes studied his high cholesterol patients, none of them experienced a heart attack. The same number of individuals, matched for age and sex in the Framingham study, experienced 54 heart attacks during that same time frame. [59] Dr. Barnes did other studies with thyroid on patients who had underlying heart disease and came to the conclusion that he was able to prevent nearly 95% of heart attacks by having his

---

[58]Leslie J Degroot; **The Thyroid and Its Disease**; Churchill Lingston, 6th Edition, 1996.

[59]Broda O. Barnes MD; **Prevention and Treatment of Coronary Heart Disease**; American Medical Association, November, 1961.

patients on thyroid. These results did not come from any selection bias in the patients in his studies. He looked at former hypothyroid patients, patients that other doctors had taken off the thyroid he recommended---taken off on the basis of normal blood tests while ignoring the basal temperature and symptom clusters. **These individuals had a very high incidence of heart attacks, much higher than seen in the general population, heart attacks often occurring within a few months of being taken off the thyroid.** That these results should have been expected was seen in 1938 throughTurner's early work with rabbits. Giving rabbits a diet that was high in cholesterol would produce arteriosclerosis, particularly if the rabbits were hypothyroid. Thyroid replacement therapy eliminated arteriosclerosis in these rabbits.[60]

The history of the use of thyroid in heart disease goes back to the early days of thyroid hormone replacement. Since thyroid helped the body get rid of excess fluid (diuretic action), it was used with good results in congestive heart failure, in which patients have fluid retention. It predated the diuretics available in medicine today. It is now known that hypothyroidism can be the sole cause of heart failure in some individuals, and this type of congestive failure will only respond to thyroid replacement therapy. The clinical recommendation given in congestive heart failure is to start the patient at ½ gr. of thyroid and increase the dosage, gradually, by 1/4 gr. at a time no more often than every two weeks.

There are always some individuals, even doctors, who do not follow instructions well. *Some doctors in the 1930s when this therapy was at its height, put patients on starting doses of thyroid well over five grains, the amount of thyroid the gland normally puts out.* In fact dosages up to 30 grainss. a day were given, six times as much thyroid as the thyroid normally produces. That kind of starting thyroid dose was deadly in some of these patients with underlying heart disease. A few patients were killed by this high starting dosage. Reports of several of these patients were collected and published in the medical literature. The impression given by these articles was that thyroid is dangerous to use in congestive heart failure and in other types of heart disease. **The myth that thyroid was dangerous to the heart had begun.**[61]

---

[60]KE Turner, CH Pressent, WH Didwell; **The Role of Thyroid in the Regulation of Blood Cholesterol in Rabbits;** Journal of Experimental Medicine, Vol 67 pp 111, 1938.

[61] Broda O Barnes MD, Charlotte Barnes; **Solved the Riddle of Heart Disease**, Robinson Press, 1976.

The experience of palpitations in hyperthyroidism---the over production of thyroid hormone---and the fact that individuals could develop palpitations on thyroid replacement added fuel to the fire, *even though palpitations are common in hypothyroidism and these palpitations go away on thyroid therapy.* It was found that in hyperthyroidism, though angina or heart pain is severe, heart attacks paradoxically are rare. This finding was ignored. The focus in hyperthyroidism was on the fact that atrial fibrillation occurs frequently. Yet even with atrial fibrillation many individuals live normal lives; live for many years without complications, though it is important to correct hyperthyroidism to try to control the fibrillation. Also ignored was the fact that low adrenal function will bring on palpitations. And in hyperthyroidism a relative adrenal deficiency is being created---the body is trying to burn more fuel than the adrenal glands are supplying. This relative deficiency may underlie the arrhythmia seen in hyperthyroidism.

The final blow to thyroid's reputation in heart disease occurred in the 1960s. A double blind study was started using thyroid hormone in heart patients, along with certain other cholesterol lowering preparations, to see which preparations would have a significant effect in lowering cholesterol and prolonging life. Unfortunately a daily dosage of 4 ½ grains. of thyroid was chosen for this study, nearly a maximum physiologic dose. Apparently the researchers felt it was too difficult to start with a small dose and increase it over time in a double blind study. The warning against starting heart patients on large doses was ignored. The researchers soon discovered for themselves that you cannot start heart patients on this kind of dose. Too many patients in the study were dying, so the code was broken. It was discovered that the patients who were receiving the thyroid hormones were dying. From the early days of experimentation on thyroid, it has been known that heart patients should not be started on a thyroid dosage greater than ½ gr. and should be increased at a pace no greater than 1/2 gr. every two weeks. The way the study was set up was a recipe for disaster. Unfortunately, the knowledge of the usefulness of thyroid hormones in heart disease was blocked by these tragic results. The true benefits of small doses of thyroid in heart patients were not brought to light.[62] It takes about two years on thyroid to gain the full protection that is available from the thyroid hormone.

Let us return to heart disease as a model and try to understand why T3-containing preparations are such an effective therapy in this disease, more effective

---

[62]Broda O Barnes MD, Charlotte Barnes; **Solved the Riddle of Heart Disease,** Robinson Press, 1976.

than can be explained just from the effects of thyroid hormones in the lowering of cholesterol level. Cholesterol is a latecomer in the damage caused by arteriosclerosis. The progressive damage is initiated by injury to blood vessel walls. Platelets congregate at the site of any vascular injury and try to repair that damage. Only if these repairs are insufficient is cholesterol brought into the picture. Thyroid tends to make platelets less sticky, so not as great a build up of platelets occurs in the repair process and the whole process of damage control is more efficient. Even after full blown arteriosclerosis is present, platelet clots play a significant role in bringing on heart attacks in the damaged coronary arteries. These platelet clots tend to be prevented by thyroid.

Recently it has been discovered that low-grade infections, often by chlamydia---organisms between a bacteria and virus in complexity---or H. pylori---the bacterium which causes peptic ulcers---also may play a role in heart attacks. An inflammation of the heart vessels caused by these organisms aggravates the tendency to form clots in the vessels. This also explains the relationship between pyrrhea or gum disease and heart attacks, for infected gums send out showers of bacteria which have been shown to infect blood vessels. Thyroid, by increasing the strength of the immune system, may prevent this low grade infection of the coronary vessels which in turn protects against heart attacks.

Thyroid also plays a significant role in vascular disease through its effects on blood pressure. At first hypothyroid patients run a low pressure, usually a systolic (the upper blood pressure number) between 100 and 110. Perhaps the low pressure is partially mediated through adrenal insufficiency which will create a low circulating blood volume through loss of salt, or sodium, which holds on to water in the body. If the blood pressure is not high enough, the blood will not be able to deliver needed nutrients to the body, so the body combats any low blood pressure through a number of different mechanisms. When blood pressure is low in the kidneys, they can't filter wastes from the body properly, so the kidneys---through a cascade of events--- produce angiotensin, a substance which raises blood pressure. Also when patients are low-thyroid, blood is shunted from the extremities into the body core, which tends to raise pressure by forcing the same volume of blood into a smaller network of vessels. This shunting is brought about by a constriction of peripheral vessels. Hypothyroid patients produce an excess of noradrenalin from the adrenal gland, which constricts blood vessels all over the body, another effort of the body to combat the low pressure. This in turn is partly related to the effort by the body to raise blood sugar levels when low. Production of Noradrenalin can actually be thirty times normal. With all this constriction of blood vessels, the blood pressure eventually reverses in hypothyroid patients and the individual becomes hypertensive after a number of years have passed. So in hypothyroidism blood pressure is either too low or too high. It is low early on, then becomes too high. If blood pressure is low, the heart tends to receive less nourishment. High blood pressure, on the other hand, damages vessel walls and initiates arteriosclerosis. In any case, the circulating blood volume is also low in hypothyroidism, and this results in the low blood pressure. Incidentally, it has been postulated recently that low circulating blood volume with the resulting stimulation of adrenalin is the underlying cause of mitral valve prolapse, a condition seen in about one in twelve individuals.

Perhaps further damage is done through a relative adrenal deficiency. Research has shown that testosterone, the male hormone, is very protective of the vascular system. Gangrene due to arteriosclerosis can be halted and healed, and abnormal EKG's in coronary artery disease can be reversed by giving individuals testosterone. The fact that the synthetic androgens used by weight lifters raise cholesterol to dangerous levels has helped block this knowledge, so most doctors consider testosterone dangerous for the heart. This is untrue and recently articles in some medical journals are recognizing this fact.

Diabetes is a good model for the effects of thyroid on the vascular system. Thyroid prevents the major problems associated with arteriosclerosis. It also prevents the ravages from micro-aneurisms occurring in small vessels which, over time, can destroy kidney tissue and eyesight. More research is needed to understand the nature of these protective effects, though the clinical evidence for this protection is strong. Perhaps elastic fibers are not being manufactured in a normal fashion leading to a weakness in the vessel walls. The vasoconstriction that takes place in hypothyroidism undoubtedly is a factor, with the resulting increase in pressure along the vessel walls tending to balloon them out into aneurisms. Perhaps homocystein---the breakdown product of the amino acid cysteine in the body---is involved. Homocystein is very damaging to vessels and is now known to be as least as great a risk factor for vascular disease as cholesterol in some individuals. The B vitamins---particularly B6, B12 and folic acid---are all critical in the metabolism of homocystein. Hypothyroidism can cause B12 deficiencies partly due to the lack of sufficient stomach acid which is known to cause B 12 deficiency. It is now known that major impairments of the nervous system from B12 deficiency can occur although the blood tests are in the normal range. Unless the other B vitamins are supplemented when thyroid is given, other deficiencies of B vitamins are also known to occur. That is why homocystein levels may be elevated in hypothyroidism.

The use of thyroid could revolutionize medicine, simply due to its effects on chronic circulatory diseases. Adequate thyroid replacement may prevent the majority of these vascular problems. Renewed research is urgently needed in this whole area.

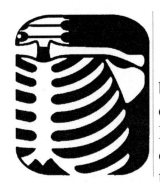

Chapter 13   The Respiratory System

Betty was tired. Some of her symptoms could be explained by a chronic anemia from a weakness of her blood vessels which often resulted in hemorrhaging. But she just did not feel good. Her skin was dry. She had a hard time sleeping. And she was cold. When diagnosed as hypothyroid and placed on replacement therapy, these nagging problems went away. Even her anemia improved as the episodes of bleeding lessened.

Though one is getting sufficient oxygen into the blood through the lungs, that oxygen needs to be carried to the individual cells of the body for proper metabolism to take place. Anemia is common in the hypothyroid patient as it was in Betty and aggravates many of the symptoms of hypothyroidism.

The effects of hypothyroidism on the respiratory system are more subtle than on other major categories of bodily function like circulation and digestion. Perhaps this is due to the fact that when the metabolism of the body is slowed, as it is in hypothyroidism, the oxygen needs of the body are lessened and the over all amount of work the respiratory system has to do is decreased. Thus the inefficiencies in this system that occur in hypothyroidism are masked. But they are important nevertheless. For there is a statistical relationship between such lung diseases as emphysema and hypothyroidism.

It is fairly common for individuals who are low thyroid to complain they feel short of breath. The oxygen saturation of their blood---the amount of oxygen being carried by the blood---is normal. However the levels of carbon dioxide (CO_2), which one might compare to exhaust fumes from the burning of glucose fuel, are slightly elevated. Since metabolism is down, these individuals should be producing less CO_2. So the body must be having a harder time getting rid of the CO_2 which is being produced. The likely explanation for this is myxedema---the polysaccharide builds up in tissue in hypothyroidism. It builds up in lung tissue as it does in other parts of the body. It then acts as a barrier for gas exchange from the capillaries in the alveoli of the lungs to the outside air. It is the rise in the levels of carbon dioxide in the bloodstream that gives hypothyroid patients the feeling of breathlessness.[63]

---

[63] Lewis E. Braverman; **Werner & Ingbar's The Thyroid**; Lippincott & Ravens Publishers 7th edition, 1996.

Of course allergies tend to be more common in hypothyroidism, partly through its effects on adrenal function. A stuffy nose from hay fever or a tightness of the airways going to the lungs in asthma will have a significant impact on breathing. The mechanisms involved have more to do with the immune system than the respiratory system and will not be considered in this chapter.

The transportation of oxygen by the blood is part of the respiratory system. Anemia, which is the lack of red blood cells or inadequate amounts of hemoglobin in these cells, decreases the ability to transport oxygen to the cells. Hypothyroidism contributes to anemia both directly and indirectly. When women are hypothyroid, their menstrual periods tend to be heavy and as a result they will often become anemic. Vitamin B12 deficiency is often severe in hypothyroidism due to lack of hydrochloric acid in the stomach, which results in lack of absorption of Vitamin B12. This in turn produces pernicious anemia, an anemia in which a decreased number of extra large red blood cells are manufactured by the marrow. This anemia lowers the ability of the blood to transport oxygen.

The production of red blood cells takes place in the marrow of long bones and is temperature dependent. This temperature dependance is clearly seen in animal models. In the tails of animals, there often is production of red blood cells in the tail bone nearest the body; but, red blood cell production quickly ceases in those bones located further from the body. Early researchers artificially warmed the tails of mice and found that the bones in the whole tail would then produce red blood cells, even those at the tip. In hypothyroidism, blood is shunted away from the extremities in order to preserve core body heat. In some individuals, the temperature in the long bones of the extremities is lowered sufficiently so that the production of red blood cells by these bones is decreased. This decreased production of red blood cells will contribute to the development of anemia, particularly if blood loss occurs for any reason. Anemia then decreases the efficiency of oxygen transport.[64]

Just a couple of other notes need to be brought out on blood and its components. The amount of thyroid hormone contained in white blood cells is quite high. Different types of white blood cells play different roles in the defenses the body has against infection. The thyroid in some of these cells may help fight infections in special ways beyond providing the increased energy needed in the battle against pathogens. But the research into these mechanisms still is preliminary. Thyroid also seems to have an

---

[64] Broda O Barnes, Lawrence Galton; **Hypothyroidism The Unsuspected Illness**, Thomas Y. Crowell Company New York, 1976.

effect on the platelets.   Blood clots do not occur as readily when thyroid function is adequate.   One might expect the opposite effect on the basis that the autonomic nervous system is geared up in hypothyroidism; it has the body ready to fight or flee. The possibility of receiving wounds means that swift clotting may be important for survival. The whole clotting mechanism is complex, so a lack of thyroid could easily cause problems in this mechanism. Wound healing which is initiated by the clotting process is definitely delayed in hypothyroidism.

In hypothyroidism the circulation tends to be sluggish, and not just in the extremities. One of the complaints individuals have who are given thyroid replacement is that their pulse becomes stronger and they often can hear their pulse beating in their ears. This unwanted noise usually fades away after a while. Blood pressure tends to be low in hypothyroidism and the vascular bed is constricted.   Later on in the course of hypothyroidism, hypertension occurs. These blood pressure factors decrease the delivery of oxygen to the cells of the body. Just the fact that metabolism is lowered in hypothyroidism indicates that cells are not utilizing the oxygen delivered to them in a normal fashion.

Normal human cells obtain most of their energy from burning glucose. The oxygen delivered to these cells is a critical part of this process. When cells become defective, they may lose their ability to burn glucose using oxygen. This is true of cancer cells. Most of their energy, like that of pathologic bacteria, comes from a fermentation process. Again, just the presence of sufficient oxygen seems to inhibit this process. After having measured the oxygen content of air trapped in ice, some researchers claim the levels of oxygen in the atmosphere have declined significantly over the past hundred years. They believe this decrease in oxygen levels is a reason for the increase in cancer and the increase in viciousness of some of the infectious diseases being seen. Other mechanism other than oxygenation may be important as well. Just the influence thyroid has on all the enzyme systems of the body should be enough reason to look at its effects more closely.   With an adequate level of thyroid on board, the body is able to remove toxins better, and the body cells tend to work efficiently and harmoniously because of the many different enzymes that are being produced in adequate amounts.

But just through its effects on oxygen delivery, thyroid likely provides some protection against cancer. There is strong anecdotal evidence that adequate thyroid replacement in hypothyroid patients can have a significant impact on the incidence of cancer. Some nutritionists who work with cancer patients report that more than ninety percent of these patients have the symptoms associated with hypothyroidism. Dr.

Barnes, in comparing his patients to the Framingham study, felt that he might be preventing nearly sixty percent of cancer by having his patients on thyroid. Certain common types of cancer were rare among his patients. For instance Dr. Barnes could not recall lung cancer developing in any of his patients that were adequately treated for hypothyroidism. Another early study looked at patients who had been treated with thyroid, then looked at the same group of patients when the doctor who cared for these patients was called up into the military for several years and these patients were taken off their thyroid therapy. Far fewer cases of cancer developed while his patients were on thyroid.

One current research project has studied strong magnetic fields in the treatment of certain cancers, such as brain cancer. Good results, even cures are reported. The studies showed these magnetic fields were greatly increasing the oxygenation of tissue, up to ten fold in some of the studies. Since historically thyroid is known to increase the oxygenation of tissue, perhaps these magnetic fields are enhancing the function of thyroid hormone in some way. This increase in oxygenation may be the mechanism behind the reports on thyroid suggesting its usefulness in cancer. Since cancer cells gain most of their energy through a fermentation process, which does not utilize oxygen, sufficient levels of thyroid will increase the likelihood of adequate oxygenation of tissues, thus possibly cutting down on the development of cancer. Little research has been done on the relationship between thyroid disease and cancer, but much more needs to be done because of the possible impact on the health of people everywhere.[65]

---

[65] Samuel Swartz BS MD; **The Relationship of Thyroid Deficiency to Cancer**; Journal of IAPM, June 1966.

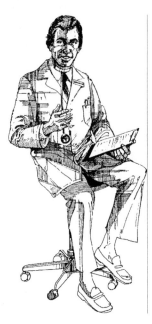

Chapter 14   Gastrointestinal Disorders

Kristie had many of the usual problems with hypothyroidism, as did many others in her family. She had allergies, frequent sinus infections and chronic headaches. She had the usual symptoms of tiredness and dry skin. But the bane of her life was diarrhea. Nothing would control the diarrhea which was threatening to take undesirable control of her life. She feared to go anywhere outside the home for fear she would not be able to make it to a rest room in time. Wearing diapers was not a viable alternative, for even these can fail. Kristie was becoming a prisoner in her own home. She was started on a combination of low dose thyroid and prednisone. The diarrhea gradually came under control as the dosage was increased. She could live again like a normal person.

Though thyroid replacement can be critical in improving digestive problems as it was in Kristie, if the body is not able to digest and absorb thyroid properly, taking thyroid will be of little use. That is one of the reasons it may take time to control the digestive symptoms which are aggravated by hypothyroidism. Hypothyroidism does have a significant impact on the whole digestive system. The formulation of Armour Thyroid was changed in the mid nineties, around 1994. The old preparation had a slightly chalky, sweet taste. The new preparation, which is supposed to break down better in the digestive system, has a medicine taste, an iodine taste to it. The old preparation was better in some ways, for all the patients could chew the tablet up, thus good absorption was virtually assured. That advice, to chew up the tablets, is no longer routinely given, for many individuals can't stand the taste. There are scattered reports of the new tablet passing through the digestive system intact. These individuals will have to chew the tablet to obtain good results.

Good absorption starts in the mouth. There food is mixed with saliva which starts the digestive process on any starches which are present. In hypothyroidism the output of saliva is often affected, and may not be produced in normal quantities. So the digestive process gets off to a poor start. Hypothyroid patients often complain about a lump in their throat with discomfort produced by swallowing. In many, this discomfort is a result of a low-grade inflammation of the thyroid gland itself. Even when the individual does not realize their thyroid gland is sore, it will give subtle symptoms in the throat, such as feeling a lump or just a need to clear the throat.

The major digestive processes start in the stomach. Its churning action thoroughly mixes all the food consumed with hydrochloric acid which the stomach secretes. In hypothyroidism, hydrochloric acid production is impaired. In fact when hypothyroidism is severe, up to fifty percent of patients have no stomach acid produced at all. If stomach acid is not present, Vitamin B12 cannot be absorbed. Therefore, one has to be alert to the possibility of a Vitamin B12 deficiency in hypothyroidism. This diagnosis can be difficult, for hypothyroidism itself causes a number of minor neurologic findings that may mimic a Vitamin B12 deficiency. When there is any question, Vitamin B12 supplementation should be given to the hypothyroid patient. Adding to the difficulty in diagnosis, some individuals will show signs of significant Vitamin B12 deficiency although their blood tests appear normal[66].

An acid environment with a pH nearly two is needed to digest protein and many complex starches properly. Rice is one of the grains that is well digested when acid is lacking and is a reason that macrobiotic diets based on rice have helped individuals with digestive problems. When food is not properly digested, gas and bloating are produced as bacteria and yeast in the intestines start fermenting the undigested food. This fermentation process can lead to diarrhea because the by- products of this process may irritate the intestines. On the other hand, in hypothyroidism the whole gastrointestinal system tends to be sluggish. Food passes through the system slowly. This in turn results in constipation which is a common finding in hypothyroidism. When waste products take longer to be eliminated from the body, bacteria have a greater chance to manufacture toxic by-products from these wastes. So there is an association of colon cancer with this constipation. The constipation also leads to the formation of diverticula or little pockets along the colon which can become infected, causing major difficulties later in life.

There is another factor at work in digestion. The absorbing surface of the intestine is a dynamic layer, operating in a harsh environment. This lining is normally completely replaced every three or four days. This replacement process takes considerable energy and will not take place completely if either thyroid function or adrenal function is too low. When this critical layer is not replaced adequately, one will see an inadequate absorbing lining produced by the intestine as the long, finger-like villae of the small intestines which provide the absorbing surface are shortened. So the body may have a difficult time absorbing the nutrition it needs for adequate function. Furthermore, partly digested protein may be able to penetrate through this

---

[66] Lewis E. Braverman; **Werner & Ingbar's The Thyroid**; Lippincott & Ravens Publishers, 7th edition, 1996.

weakened layer, leading to what is referred to as a "leaky gut" syndrome. Undigested protein molecules make their way into the blood stream. The body starts reacting to these large protein molecules as if they are foreign invaders and begins developing sensitivities to foods. Women have a more significant problem with a "leaky gut". If they are questioned closely, twenty percent will state there are some foods that bother them in some way.

Recent evidence shows giving a number of immunizations in combination, such as in the MMR vaccine, can produce an immune complex which attacks the ileum of the gut producing a "leaky gut syndrome". In severe cases this can lead to autism in children as the body begins to absorb toxins. In milder cases evidence exists that it can produce an attention deficit disorder. So unfortunately, many of the digestive problems may start in childhood.

At times just a lack of thyroid hormone may be responsible for the initiation of the whole process leading to a "leaky gut". When the leaking of protein through the gut wall is marked, these individuals may develop severe inflammatory diseases of the colon called colitis. Many with a milder problem will have irritable bowel disease with indigestion, with alternating constipation and diarrhea. At present the medical profession does a poor job controlling the conditions stemming from a "leaky gut". When the digestive system is not working properly, the problem is aggravated by the yeast, candida, and by various bacteria not usually present in the GI tract. The body has a normal intestinal flora made up of bacteria that help the body in the digestive process. Three pounds of these bacteria are present in the intestine and manufacture important substances such as Vitamin K which is involved with the clotting of blood for the body. These good bacteria can be replaced by bacteria that produce toxic substances, bacteria which in health are only present in small numbers. But these harmful bacteria can become dominant if conditions are right. All of us have experienced the ability of some of these harmful organisms to produce diarrhea, usually from the introduction of a harmful species from some outside source. Abnormal yeast infestations are likely more important than the bacteria, for yeasts are capable of producing toxins that undermine the immune system of the body and greatly increase the toxic load the body has to get rid of. These bacteria and yeast reflect our own society. The largest group in our own society is that of the hard-working tax-paying citizens. A second smaller group lives off welfare payments, off the efforts of the first, hardworking group. The smallest group is the criminal element that is actually destructive to the rest of society. Thyroid is able to keep these last two undesirable elements of the intestinal "society" under control. A milk-free, gluten-free diet is also helpful in individuals who are having these digestive problems.

When discussing the thyroid's role in digestion, obesity must be mentioned. Hypothyroidism is often associated with being overweight. There is a mismatch between the calories absorbed and those utilized, for the body is not able to burn all the calories it receives through digestion, and these extra calories are stored as fat. But there are hypothyroid individuals who are not able to absorb sufficient calories to maintain normal weight. And so they are underweight, and are not able to gain weight no matter what they do. When thyroid hormone therapy is started on individuals who are hypothyroid, one of the first effects is that digestion is improved. Even those who are overweight start absorbing calories more efficiently from the food they eat. Not only will those who are underweight start gaining, but on small doses of thyroid, about a third of those who are overweight will actually find that their weight is increasing as well. In an other third, this small weight gain is countered by the loss of the excess fluid that is retained in hypothyroidism and their weight remains unchanged on low dose thyroid hormone supplementation. Higher doses of thyroid are frequently needed to bring the body into a true balance. Doses must be increased until the metabolism of the body matches the caloric intake. Control of weight on thyroid replacement therapy occurs in about two thirds of individuals. At times, though, an individual's weight does not decrease, the body gets rid of excess fat and adds protein, so there is a change in body size though not in weight; loss of inches around the waist occurs in the absence of a weight change. A third of individuals still struggle with their weight although they are on thyroid hormones and will have to pay attention to the carbohydrate, protein balance in the foods they eat. Doing this most individuals will be able to lose their excess weight. One must remember that what nature has set as the proper body weight may not be the same as what the latest fashion magazine suggests. Even though one's weight is not fully controlled, one will usually be healthy when on adequate thyroid replacement.

Before leaving the topic of digestion, the role the liver plays needs to be mentioned. Nutrients absorbed from the intestines pass through the liver before they are sent out to the body to be used. The liver wears many hats. It will latch onto any substance that is toxic, and if it is not overworked, will eliminate that toxic substance from the body. This involves a two phase process. In the first phase, the toxin is changed, often by having an alcohol group added to it. In the second phase, the toxin is conjugated to make it more soluble so the body can get rid of it. The substance may actually become more toxic in the first step. For example, Candida in the intestines increases the amount of chemicals called aldehydes that are produced. When the liver has an excessive amount of aldehydes to process, chloral hydrate is often formed. Chloral hydrate is the main ingredient in many over the counter sleeping tablets. This is just one mechanism that can contribute to fatigue if the liver is not functioning properly.

Since the liver is such an active organ, it utilizes more thyroid hormone than any other organ does. So hypothyroidism has a major impact on liver function. For instance, when the liver is sluggish one often sees a yellowish hue to the skin. When the liver can't keep up with its workload, it isn't able to convert all the beta carotene that it receives into active Vitamin A. The buildup of beta carotene produces the yellowish hue. More importantly, as a result many individuals are deficient in Vitamin A if they are hypothyroid.

Many hypothyroid patients report that they are sensitive to medications, perhaps not being able to tolerate the full dose others seem to handle without a problem. Again, the liver is having a hard time detoxifying all these medications, a hard time in removing them from the body. So the amount of medication will build up to abnormally high levels even though individuals are given the standard dose of the medication. This results in the fact that side effects of medications are far more common when one is low thyroid, for side effects generally are much greater when the levels of medication are higher in the body. In effect, one is giving a higher dosage of medication to hypothyroid patients because their ability to get rid of the medicine is limited.

The liver also processes cholesterol. Cholesterol is turned into bile which is important in the digestion of fats by the body. This process becomes sluggish in hypothyroid individuals. Cholesterol stones form in the gall bladder. Therefore, cholecystitis, or a gall bladder attack, is a frequent complication of underlying hypothyroidism. Gall bladder surgery is a common marker for the individual with hypothyroidism. The liver itself tends to get clogged with excessive cholesterol and may not function properly unless it is cleansed.

As mentioned, the liver as the most active "factory" in the body uses large amounts of thyroid. It cannot do its job properly in the hypothyroid individual. But it also has an important role in thyroid metabolism. It shares the T3 it produces with the brain, It also is able to add a sulphur group to the thyroid molecule, transforming it so it can be eliminated in the bile. Bacteria in the intestine can strip this sulphur group off the thyroid molecule, rejuvenating it, thus the body can reabsorb active thyroid hormones, which can be reused. Digestive problems influence this reabsorption of thyroid---constipation will increase the reabsorption while diarrhea will decrease the reabsorption. The hypothyroid patient gets an additional supply of thyroid, while the hyperthyroid patient who will tend toward diarrhea will get rid of more thyroid helping bring the system in balance.[67]

The effects of thyroid on the digestive system make a major contribution to the maintenance of good health.

[67]Sing-yung Wu, Theo J Vissar; **Thyroid Hormone Metabolism-Molecular Biology**; CRC Press, 1994.

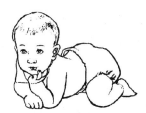

Chapter 15   The Nervous System

Joseph was born with Down's syndrome. He spent much of his first year in and out of the hospital. Then he was started on thyroid supplementation and on low dose steroids. He did not need to be hospitalized again until he was four years old.   At that time, asthma---complicating respiratory infections---necessitated re-hospitalization. But over all he was doing well. He was strong and active, and was making good progress mentally for a Down's child.

The basal metabolism test showed that all Down's children are hypothyroid like Joseph. This truth was forgotten with the advent of the blood tests for thyroid. Other children may be born with even more serious thyroid problems. About one child in four thousand is born without a functioning thyroid gland. It is routine to screen newborn infants for their thyroid function, for if infants with severe hypothyroidism are missed, if they are not given thyroid replacement therapy, lack of thyroid will produce what is termed cretinism. Cretins are mentally retarded, are short in stature, have large tongues---appear very much like those with Down's syndrome. Thyroid is critical to normal brain development. The circulating levels of thyroid in a newborn are much higher than the levels in adults---up to sixteen times higher. In fact on a weight basis, newborns who lack thyroid function are given a thyroid dosage that is ten times higher than the dosage given an adult. And even in a ten-year-old child, the amount of thyroid produced per pound body weight can still be twice as much as an adult will produce. The adrenal hormone levels are also much higher than in an adult---pregnenolone levels are up to twenty times higher. It make one wonder if thyroid and adrenal were used together in large doses if some of the mental deterioration seen in aging could be reversed but at this time no experiments have been done, even in animal models. We do know thyroid is critical for mental development.

Experiments on rats have indicated that the longer an embryonic animal is without thyroid the worse the mental problems. The earlier this deprivation occurs, the worse the problems seen in the brain. So it is critical for replacement therapy of thyroid to be begun early. If a child lacking thyroid is more than four months old when replacement therapy is initiated, some mental retardation will definitely occur. In fact, therapy should be initiated before the child is three months of age in order to guarantee the child will function in a fashion that is nearly normal.[68]

---

[68]Gernard Labra, Alan Belanex et. al.; **Neonatal Thyroid Screening**, Raven Press NY, 1980.

Other studies have indicated the importance of thyroid in brain development. In the sixties a group of retarded children, many of them with Down's syndrome, were given vitamin, mineral and thyroid therapy in an effort to improve their mental functioning. Their subsequent mental development was followed and measured with standard intelligence tests. These children were able to increase their IQs by an average of twenty points, to a level at which they were able to meet their own basic needs and to cope with simple society. One child, who was about seven years of age when the study began, initially scored around 30 for his mental age on his tests, a level of function comparable to that of a baby. Two years later after being on thyroid, vitamins and minerals, he had learned to read and scored in the normal range on his I.Q. tests. Unfortunately these promising results do not seem to have been followed up in other studies.

Thyroid affects the developing brain in other ways as well. When thyroid is lacking it is not just the neurons that don't develop well, the structural cells---the supporting architecture of the brain---does not develop adequately either. When thyroid levels have been low in the developing brain, the individual is prone to have seizures. Some of the protective insulating features of the brain have been lost. If thyroid therapy is not started soon enough in those who would become cretins, fully twenty percent of these individuals will have a significant seizure problem. No study seems to have looked at individuals who have seizures to investigate what percentage of these patients have hypothyroid symptoms. Anecdotal evidence would indicate that seizure patients often do have signs of being low thyroid. Petit mal seizures, those in which there is a momentary loss of consciousness, also seem to have a relationship to hypoglycemia. So treating hypothyroidism may have a direct effect in helping these individuals through helping control their blood sugar levels.[69]

Adults also have problems with their brains if thyroid function is low. They have a hard time concentrating, short term memory often becomes poor, and it may be difficult for them to find the right word to use when talking or they may have difficulty pronouncing that word correctly. Hypothyroid individuals frequently become nervous and irritable. Depression is extremely common and should always call for an evaluation for possible hypothyroidism. Psychiatrists have discovered that in depressed patients when the usual antidepressants are not working, adding thyroid will frequently restore the effectiveness of the antidepressants. In fact often thyroid by itself will get rid of depression. They have found that Synthroid, a pure T4 preparation, does not work. These individuals need T3 in order to get rid of their symptoms. The reason

---

[69] Leslie J Degroot; **The Thyroid and Its Diseases**, Churchhill, Lingnstorn 6th ed., 1996.

for this goes back to the fact that the conversion of T4 to T3 is catalyzed in most parts of the brain by a type II de-iodinase. This enzyme is actually inhibited by T4---extra amounts of T4 decrease the production of T3 in the brain cells. So it is easy to understand why T3 would be much more effective in this situation. In this regard it is also interesting that the glucocorticoids greatly enhance the conversion of T4 to T3 in the brain. It is well known that some of the adrenal hormones will increase concentration and memory. It is also well known that larger doses of glucocorticoids can produce a feeling of euphoria, or extreme well being. The problem with these high doses is that while the function of the brain is being enhanced, the same cortisone dosage is shutting down the metabolism of the rest of the body. The right dosage of steroids, a physiologic dosage, is extremely important. Steroids in low doses may be helpful in many mental conditions and research needs to be conducted in order to discover just what role these medications might be able to play when balanced with thyroid.

More serious mental problems are associated with low thyroid as well. Hypothyroidism can produce all the symptoms of mental illness---not just depression. Individuals who are severely hypothyroid often develop hallucinations and delusions of various sorts. When thyroid function is totally absent, studies done before thyroid replacement was available showed that half these severe myxedema patients developed psychotic symptoms. In many mental diseases, hypothyroidism may be a contributing factor. For example, it is known that many patients with manic-depression are extremely sensitive to low blood-glucose levels. A five-hour glucose tolerance test which gives a large sugar load to those being tested will call forth many of the manic symptoms these individuals suffer from, as sugar levels drop due to an overproduction of insulin. Since thyroid controls the utilization of glucose by the cells, thyroid hormone has a significant effect on these patients. Many of these same individuals might benefit from adrenal support as well. Lithium, which is often used to treat manic-depressive patients, blocks thyroid function and careful attention to thyroid function is needed in these individuals. Most will develop signs of hypothyroidism if they do not have such signs already. [70]

It is not just the central nervous system that is affected by hypothyroidism. The peripheral nerves are affected as well. Three different patterns are seen in the peripheral nerves. At times a generalized degeneration of the nerves is observed. More commonly pigment is laid down in the nerve bundles which decreases the

---

[70]J. H. Lazarus, R. John et. al.; **Lithium Therapy and Thyroid**; Psychol. Med. V.11 pp. 85-92, 1981.

efficiency of function of the same nerves. But the most common problem is related to myxedema---the mucous material that collects in the tissues.   The mucous material collects around the nerves and swells as these polysaccharides hold on to water. This puts pressure on the nerves.   When the nerves pass through narrow spaces, this pressure becomes important. This seems to be the mechanism behind the increased incidence of carpal tunnel syndrome in hypothyroid patients, a situation where the median nerve is pinched in the hand near the wrist, giving rise to numbness in the fingers.

It is common to have sensations in the peripheral nerves in hypothyroidism---tingling and crawling sensations in the skin. In fact, nearly eighty percent of hypothyroid patients report such problems. Which of the mechanisms underlie these sensations has not been clearly elucidated. It may simply involve nutrition to the nerves or the sluggish metabolism of the nerves in hypothyroidism. In other individuals one will see restless legs, symptoms which frequently go away with thyroid replacement therapy.

All parts of the nervous system are affected. The autonomic nervous system does not escape unscathed. In hypothyroid patients, the autonomic nervous system is stimulated---the body is prepared for fight or flight. In the attempt of the body to control hypoglycemia the levels of norepinephrine may climb to 30 times higher than normal. These high levels have an impact on these individuals. In children one often sees agitation, inability to concentrate for more than a moment, and hyperactivity. It is less common to see this pattern in an adult. This over stimulation of the autonomic nervous system is balanced by the fact that these individuals lack energy. Most adults who are hypothyroid just do not have enough energy to express the inner feeling of nervousness. But many of them when questioned relay the fact they often feel keyed up but give no outward expression of this. Children are more apt to express the inner tension outwardly resulting in hyperactive behavior.

When hypothyroid patients develop hypotension, the drugs used to raise blood pressure often do not work well. This is because the blood vessels are already clamped down through the actions of the autonomic nervous system and medications will not produce any further constriction of the vessels.   In these patients replacement of adequate fluid volume is key. This is particularly true in patients who have severe hypothyroidism. This fact is important to keep in mind in the treatment of shock.

In summary, both thyroid and adrenal hormones have critical roles to play in the functioning of the nervous system.   More attention needs to be paid to their role in nervous system disorders.

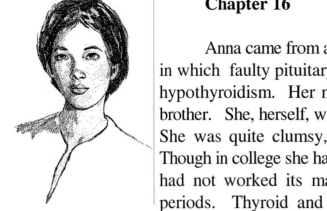

Chapter 16   Exclusively Female

Anna came from a secondary hypothyroid family, a family in which faulty pituitary function seemed to be the cause of the hypothyroidism. Her mother was hypothyroid and so was her brother. She, herself, was tired, had dry skin, and retained fluid. She was quite clumsy, easily able to trip over her own feet. Though in college she had a young, girlish appearance. Estrogen had not worked its magic on her and she had no menstrual periods. Thyroid and adrenal replacement therapy gradually began their work in her, and her concentration and sluggishness improved. Finally after three years, as a college graduate, she was introduced to the 'wonders of womanhood'.

Just as testosterone, an adrenal type hormone, controls the sexual characteristics such as beard and muscle strength of the male, so the sexual characteristics in the female are controlled by another adrenal type hormone, estrogen. Though these hormones are produced by the testes and ovaries, significant amounts are produced by the adrenal gland. When the adrenal glands don't produce sufficient sex hormones, this lack can have an enormous effect on the menstrual cycle as it did in Anna.

Actually men need some estrogen and women some testosterone, but in much smaller amounts than is necessary for the opposite sex for certain vital functions in the body. The control of estrogen in the female is more complex than the control of testosterone in the male, for the levels of estrogen change markedly during the menstrual cycle. And as mentioned elsewhere, there is a close relationship between the binding sites of thyroid and the binding sites of estrogen, so the function of thyroid and estrogen are intertwined in subtle ways. Women are several times more likely than men to complain of symptoms relating to hypothyroidism as a result of these interrelated binding sites.[71]

The female menstrual cycle is under the control of pituitary hormones. One is follicle stimulating hormone, FSH, which among other things matures the eggs in the ovary and prepares an egg to be released each month during the menstruating years. Prolactin, another pituitary hormone is also involved. Its most visible function involves milk production. Thyroid hormones do have an effect on these hormone systems, but

---

[71]E. Roderick, M. Scott et .al.; **Interactions of Estrogen and Thyroid Hormone Receptors**; Neurobiology and Behavior, II-11, pp 1581-1592, Oct 1997.

the clinical impact is far less than the impact that thyroid hormones have on estrogen. This chapter will concentrate on estrogen and progesterone, though Prolactin and FSH both have important roles. A lack of these hormones in hypothyroidism contributes to the delay in the development of a normal menstrual cycle in girls and also to the delay of associated secondary sexual characteristics.

Not only will menstrual cycles be delayed in hypothyroid individuals, they are often irregular. But worse, periods tend to be heavy and painful. These individuals also frequently have PMS or premenstrual tension, sometimes to an extent that is incapacitating. Often the menstrual bleeding associated with hypothyroidism is difficult to control and many women wind up on birth control pills in an effort to control this bleeding. At times even the birth control pills are not successful, so frequent D&C procedures become part of the experience of these women. Too often they eventually wind up with hysterectomies to bring this bleeding problem under control---a problem that could have been corrected with a little thyroid replacement therapy and perhaps a little adrenal support for balance.

But menstrual irregularities are not the only harmful effect thyroid has on the uterus. A lack of thyroid greatly enhances the growth of **uterine fibroids** as well. If a woman is on sufficient amounts of thyroid the further growth of uterine fibroids usually will be blocked and frequently they will start shrinking. Besides uncontrolled bleeding, the major reason that women have hysterectomies is symptomatic uterine fibroids which can cause discomfort and contribute to excessive bleeding.[72] Hypothyroidism also increases the incidence of uterine cancer which is the reason behind most of the remaining hysterectomies. (The relationship between hypothyroidism and cancer was dealt with in another chapter.) So thyroid has an almost magical impact on many of the woes associated with womanhood; it takes them away.

This includes a decrease in all types of **vaginitis**, the infections peculiar to women. Thyroid increases the resistance of the body to all types of infection. The repeated yeast infections some women experience often improve greatly, and other types of vaginitis are decreased as well. Repeated urinary tract infections are another significant problem that some women find often clear up with thyroid therapy. A urinary tract infection is one of the commonest reasons women seek medical help.

---

[72] Broda O. Barnes MD, Lawrence Galton; **Hypothyroidism, the Unsuspected Illness**; Thomas Y Crowell Company, New York, 1976.

Thyroid therapy does not mean one is free to ignore common sense. Adequate thyroid therapy will not prevent sexually transmitted diseases, though their severity will often be lessened and the severe complications may be avoided. Avoiding exposure is by far the most important thing anyone can do.

All portions of the female anatomy are impacted by thyroid hormone. The breasts certainly are. **Fibrocystic disease** of the breast is far more common in hypothyroidism. So just being on thyroid will tend to prevent breast lumps that need to be biopsied. Taking sufficient vitamin E and avoiding too much caffeine are also very important in this regard. If women will do all three, they will prevent a majority of the breast's problems that plague them. And of course, the increased strength of the immune system while on sufficient thyroid will tend to prevent mastoiditis or breast infections.

The lactating breast is also impacted. Hypothyroidism can be the cause of insufficient milk production in the young mother. If a woman is having problems breast-feeding her child, her thyroid function should be checked. Thyroid replacement therapy will often return the milk production to normal.

Before leaving breast problems, let me add that an excess of estrogen increases the lumpiness of the breasts. Estrogen stimulates the growth of breast tissue. Many women are afraid of estrogen replacement therapy because they fear that this may increase the incidence of breast cancer. The secret of good health lies in balance. If dosages of estrogen are too large, they will produce side effects. Except for hot flashes, the other symptoms of menopause including the prevention of bone loss can be controlled with doses of estrogen that will not increase cancer risks, doses that are smaller than are usually given in estrogen replacement therapy. Estrogen also has a significant impact in women, just in their ability to think clearly and is needed in small doses in menopausal women. Since natural progesterone will greatly enhance bone strength and will mitigate against the unwanted effects of estrogen, these hormones need to be given together and are important in the balance leading to health.

The topic of pregnancy will be considered next. In a previous generation, doctors often gave women thyroid hormone if they were having difficulty becoming pregnant These doctors knew taking additional thyroid often worked but they did not know why. We can still only guess at the reason. Estrogen sharpens the body's ability to recognize any substance that is foreign to it. We mentioned that autoimmune disorders are more common in women for this reason. When an excess of estrogen is present, the estrogen responds to the newly fertilized egg that tries to implant in the uterus as a foreign invader, destroying it. Progesterone is needed, for the progesterone blunts this estrogen response. Thus the progesterone protects the fertilized egg and allows the early embryo to implant in the uterus. As pregnancy progresses, large amounts of estrogen and progesterone are produced. The progesterone is needed at all times to counter the effects of the estrogen. Both these hormones are likely important for normal development of the fetus. There is some evidence for example that extra progesterone around the third and fourth months of pregnancy will enhance the intelligence of the child. And thyroid certainly has a significant impact on the normal development of the fetus and on the whole course of pregnancy. [73]

One of the clinical observations of Dr. Barnes was that when mothers were hypothyroid, they tended to give birth to large babies. In fact he discovered that a birth weight of eight pounds in a first child was an almost sure indicator of hypothyroidism in the mother. Usually large babies are connected with being pre-diabetic. This relationship to hypothyroidism is largely unappreciated.

Perhaps the most tragic effect of hypothyroidism in pregnancy is the frequent occurrence of miscarriages. Spontaneous abortion is far more common when mothers are hypothyroid. Any time spontaneous abortion occurs, hypothyroidism must be suspected. And when repeated abortions occur, hypothyroidism is almost always an underlying cause.

Another condition that has long been known to have a strong relationship to hypothyroidism is toxemia of pregnancy. This life-threatening situation is one in which the mother develops massive fluid retention and severe hypertension toward the end of pregnancy. It is far more common in hypothyroidism. Adequate thyroid replacement therapy should prevent most cases, and if toxemia does occur it should be much milder.

Thyroid may make other contributions to an uneventful pregnancy as well. A family practitioner in Idaho, after observing the effects of thyroid in his patients, placed all his pregnant patients on thyroid, some four hundred individuals altogether. He found that by doing so he was able to prevent premature labor. The usual incidence of premature labor is a little more than ten percent. He had two cases of premature labor in his patients---a twenty-times lesser incidence than is usually seen. Both these women had other significant underlying reasons why they went into premature labor.

---

[73]Lewis E. Braverman; **Werner & Ingbar's The Thyroid**, Lippincott & Ravens Publishers 7th edition, 1996.

One of them had an incompetent cervix, a condition that brings on very early labor. And the other had what is called a bicornate uterus, a congenital abnormality that often does not allow room for a fetus to grow to maturity.

So by using thyroid, this doctor was able to nearly eliminate the heartache associated with the birth of premature infants. He further observed that in the offspring of these mothers he seemed to have eliminated most mental developmental difficulties such as attention deficit disorder; but he had not studied these children closely enough to be sure that his observations were true. It is a known fact, though, that in pregnancy, the health of both mother and child is affected by lack of thyroid.

Thyroid profoundly affects females in all stages of their lives, particularly during the reproductive years when estrogen is produced in large quantities. Sufficient thyroid can greatly increase the quality of life for women by its impact during this time. And as thyroid seems to enhance libido, it will increase the enjoyment of womanhood in more subtle ways---not only in physical well-being, but in mental well-being as well. More research is needed to discover the full potential thyroid replacement has for women.

\

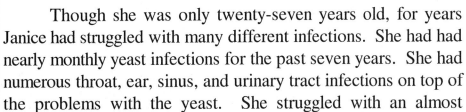

Chapter 17   INFECTIONS

Though she was only twenty-seven years old, for years Janice had struggled with many different infections. She had had nearly monthly yeast infections for the past seven years. She had numerous throat, ear, sinus, and urinary tract infections on top of the problems with the yeast. She struggled with an almost unbearable tiredness, needing naps of up to three hours in the afternoon in order to function. Also every time she bent down to do anything she would feel dizzy and would have to stand still until the spinning stopped. She dreaded having to stoop down for any reason, even to play with her children, for along with the dizziness would come severe headaches. These problems made it almost impossible for Janice to keep up with her children and household chores. She had consulted many different doctors who had run a variety of tests, all reported back as normal. When she was finally diagnosed as hypothyroid, she was placed on Westhroid and her symptoms gradually went away. She still has a cold or sore throat now and then like everyone else, but her health has been restored to normal.

Infections often run rampant when an individual like Janice has hypothyroidism. This has been known from the earliest days of research on the thyroid gland. Some of the reasons for this relationship are just beginning to be understood. Dr. Broda Barnes carefully studied the relationship between tuberculosis and hypothyroidism. He went to Bavaria every year to a city that by law had autopsies done on everyone who died in that city. On the basis of his findings, he developed the thesis that in the previous generation those who had died of TB and other infectious diseases were now living long enough to die of chronic diseases, like heart disease and cancer instead. [74]

All too soon the problems that previous generations faced are forgotten. In the mid 1800s the most common cause of death was tuberculosis. On death certificates, well over one quarter of deaths were charged to this one disease. Other infectious diseases also took their toll, killing many more---in fact few families were untouched by early death from infectious disease a hundred years ago. For example, those with TB seldom lived past their early thirties, dying a full decade before the signs of heart disease appear. The population that was susceptible to heart disease was dying off before heart disease could develop. Even today TB remains a scourge in developing countries; in these areas TB is still the biggest killer of young women in their child-

---

[74] Broda O Barnes MD, Lawrence Galton; **Hypothyroidism, the Unsuspected Illness,** Thomas Y Crowell Company, New York, 1976.

bearing years.

Some of the early researchers in thyroid demonstrated clearly that hypothyroidism has a profound effect on the immune system and thus on the ability of the body to fight off disease. But they had no real understanding of why this was so. For example, experimental animals were infected with tuberculosis. (Much of this research was done on rabbits.) The thyroid glands of these animals were removed and different thyroid replacement dosage schedules were given to these animals from doses low enough to create severe hypothyroidism to high doses creating hyperthyroidism. The researchers discovered that the worse the hypothyroidism, the worse the prognosis due to the TB infecting these animals. Animals in each dosage range were sacrificed and the severity of the disease measured through autopsy findings. The worst manifestations of tuberculosis are generally found in the lungs. The researchers found a straight line response or a direct correlation between the severity of the lung disease and lack of thyroid hormone. When these experimental animals had little thyroid, the lesions in the lungs were large and teeming with TB bacteria. As the dosage of thyroid was increased, these lesions shrank in size and contained fewer bacteria. In the hyperthyroid animal, the lesion became small and contained relatively few bacteria. (Billions of bacteria were still present.) But compared to the hypothyroid rabbits, those in the hyperthyroid range actually had a thousand times fewer TB bacteria and the animal's own defense systems were able to control these lesser infestations. Overwhelming infections were only seen in hypothyroid animals. The defenses of the body were able to handle the onslaught of tuberculosis far better if the animals had normal thyroid function.

If an individual's thyroid function is normal, it is unlikely they will come down with TB. On the other hand, individuals who contract TB are usually hypothyroid. Therefore, thyroid hormones should hold a very important place in the treatment of this disease. In the usual patient with tuberculosis, among the trillions of invading organisms, half a dozen possess a natural immunity to any single antibiotic that might be used to treat his or her TB. The most important medication in the treatment is INH---isoniazide. In addition to INH, another medication, (often rifampin in the USA today) has to be given so resistant TB does not develop. If the second drug is not given, those TB organisms with natural resistance to the antibiotic will multiply and take over the infection. INH is cheap; other TB medications are not. So developing countries have a hard time treating their tuberculosis population adequately. It is just too expensive to give the second drug. If the number of organisms could be decreased a thousand-fold with the use of relatively cheap thyroid, it might be possible to treat these patients with the single medication, INH, making the treatment of TB affordable in developing countries. This might save the lives of many young women.

Why is thyroid important for the immune system as it fights infectious diseases? More than one answer is starting to emerge. The most basic one may simply be that the body needs energy to fight bacterial and viral invaders, and in hypothyroid states not enough energy is available for the battle. It is now known that the output of adrenal glucocorticoids is increased six-fold in response to many infections.[75] It is logical that there is a corresponding increase in thyroid to help burn the extra fuel that the body is releasing from its stores. Among its other properties, thyroid does enhance the entry of glucose into the cells where it can be utilized. Some recent research indicates that influenza organisms freeze the production of the glucocorticoids before the victims come down with their flu symptoms. Flu is actually uncommon when thyroid levels in the body are adequate, and when flu does occur it tends to be mild. Again balance between the thyroid and adrenal hormones is important, as well as the total amounts of these hormones. Many bacterial invaders use glucose as an energy source and if more is produced than the body is able to utilize, the invaders are helped by being given a plentiful energy source and resistance of the body is decreased---the situation seen in diabetes where glucose levels are too high since the glucose is not being utilized properly. Thus, infections in diabetics tend to be more severe.

Most pathologic bacteria are anaerobic---they use a fermentation process to produce their energy. These fermentation processes tend to be shut down in the presence of oxygen. Just the fact that thyroid tends to increase the oxygen supply to the tissues through improved circulation keeps the severity of many of these infections in check. This is particularly true of infections of the skin where decreased circulation to the extremities and skin greatly increases the susceptibility to superficial skin infections.

Frequent infections of any kind are often a signal that thyroid function is not adequate. This is first seen in young children with frequent infections occurring from a variety of causes. More indicative of hypothyroidism are such problems as chronic ear infections and frequent bouts of pharyngitis or sore throats. Chronic sinus infections run hand-in-hand with hypothyroidism. In fact, the majority of hypothyroid patients seen in the Rocky Mountain region have at least a mild chronic sinus condition, the reason Dr. Barnes used an axillary temperature to measure basal temperature. Repeated urinary tract infections are associated with hypothyroidism and usually go away with thyroid replacement therapy. But perhaps an even more important signal of

---

[75]William McK Jeffries; **Safe Uses of Cortisone**, 1994.

hypothyroidism is the occurrence of any severe infection. For example, pneumonia is rare when individuals have normal thyroid function. Following any severe infection, thyroid status should be investigated.

Recently another possible role that thyroid may play in fighting infections has been uncovered. Many white blood cells are high in thyroid content. White blood cells are attracted to the site of an infection. As shown earlier, the thyroid molecule has two rings both with two iodide atoms attached. In the white blood cells the body is able to split the linkage between these two rings. When it does so, free iodine is released. Iodine is a very active molecule. The body directs the iodine against the invading organisms. It is able to latch onto them and helps kill them. Iodine is a common skin antiseptic, and it seems the body is using iodine in the same fashion against invading bacteria and virus.

It is well known that illness of any kind can have a profound effect on thyroid functioning. This condition with abnormal blood tests, usually low T3 levels , is often termed Non-Thyroid Illness or the Euthyroid Sick Syndrome by the medical profession. Since blood tests usually gradually revert to normal when the underlying illness is past, the thyroid abnormalities produced in these conditions have not been considered to be true thyroid problems. But the underlying transformation of T4 to T3 in the cells may not return to normal. Adding to this false understanding of on Non- Thyroid illness, when thyroid has been given to these patients when they are ill, most of the time it has not helped. Let us try to understand clearly what is happening. Anything that will interfere with the fuel supply of the cells will affect thyroid functioning. An inadequate fuel supply shuts down metabolism. In fever, if an inadequate amount of glucose is being supplied to meet the energy needs of a cell, the cell will decrease its T3 output along with its rate of metabolism. In other types of illness, say in shock where decreased circulation slows glucose transport, the body is not able to provide adequate amounts of glucose to the cells, so the cells again reign in their metabolism by producing less T3. Often under these conditions, when thyroid has been tried, a synthetic T4 preparation like synthroid has been given. Since the formation of T3 from T4 is blocked when the fuel supply is inadequate, giving T4 will have little effect on the course of events; T4 itself has limited potency, thus showing no effectiveness. Giving a T3 preparation may be even worse for the individual, for that will force the cells to burn up more fuel supplies than they actually have, resulting in further injury to these cells. Only when the fuel supply is restored to the cells can the metabolism be increased safely. Only then will thyroid be beneficial. It is interesting that the glucocorticoids, hormones which tap the body's energy stores, have often been used and have been found helpful in Non-Thyroid Illness. When a patient is in shock, for example, the underlying shock must be treated first so the fuel supply to the cells is reestablished. Then it becomes proper to increase the metabolism of the cells by increasing the thyroid, by means of a T3 containing preparation. Then thyroid indeed will be found to be beneficial, and Non-Thyroid Illness will be seen to be a significant cause of thyroid problems that should be addressed by the medical profession.

AIDS infection with its profound effect on the immune system is a special case with a unique effect on thyroid function. Researchers have discovered that the AIDS virus uses selenium in its reproductive cycle. It has such a high affinity for the selenium that it steals selenium from the body's enzymes of those infected with the virus. The symptoms of severe selenium deficiency parallel those of the AIDS virus. Two of the three known de-iodinase that regulate T4 to T3 and T4 to RT3 conversions in the cell are selenium-containing enzymes. Although the body protects these thyroid regulating molecules at the expense of other selenium containing enzymes in the human body, devastation of thyroid function still seems to occur. If individuals cannot produce T3 from T4, they become functionally hypothyroid. Since this type of hypothyroid problem is not picked up on the currently used blood tests, the poor thyroid function is not suspected. Hypothyroidism created by selenium deficiency is contributing to the woes of AIDS patients. They have decreased metabolism in their tissues and do not have sufficient energy available to fight off the AIDS virus. It is probable that thyroid will be found to be very beneficial in the treatment of these patients.

Today medicine is facing a new reign of terror from infectious diseases as antibiotics seem to have less and less ability to cope with the resistant strains that are emerging. The proper use of thyroid may prove to be one of the most important weapons in the battle and may turn the tide to victory over infectious disease.

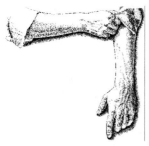

Chapter 18   Skin Conditions

Al was adopted, so no medical family history was known to his parents. However, it was all too evident that he had significant health problems. From the time he came to his new home as a baby, he had severe eczema. Every part of his body was covered with rash. Special formulas gave little relief. He had frequent upper respiratory infections as well. As a three year old toddler, the rash was just as bad. He would scratch himself to sleep each night, at times until his skin was actually bleeding. He also had a short attention span and was constantly on the go. He would not stop long enough to listen to his mother read a book. Just the severe eczema in this child gave a strong suspicion of hypothyroidism. But coupled with a low basal temperature and his other symptoms the presence of hypothyroidism was certain, so it was elected to treat him with thyroid hormones. When he was placed on thyroid, he became a different child. He would sit and listen to his mother read, showing a decent attention span. The eczema gradually improved to the point it was no longer a major problem.

Once crude desiccated thyroid preparations became available, they were tried on individuals with skin rashes to see if the thyroid would help get rid of these troublesome conditions. In 1893 an English physician by the name of Dr. B. Branwell reported spectacular results on a variety of skin problems as did some other doctors in Europe. Unfortunately when doctors in the United States repeated these experiments, the thyroid preparations then available to them were so weak they observed little or no effect. So unlike Al, these patients did not respond to their treatment. When more potent preparations became available, these experiments unfortunately were not repeated---it was not until 1915 that consistently potent preparations became available. So the profound effect that hypothyroidism has on skin disease was never clearly understood in the United States. Thyroid was not brought into the arsenal of dermatology, the study and treatment of skin disease.

Let us look briefly at the effect hypothyroidism has on the skin. When thyroid production is insufficient to maintain the metabolism of the whole body, the body still tries to maintain the metabolism of its essential systems. These include the functioning of various internal organs such as the liver and kidneys. In order to preserve the core body temperature so these organs will function efficiently enough to maintain the body's essential functions, blood is shunted away from the skin and the extremities. There are small structures, the globus, which are gatekeepers in the vascular system. Their job is to shunt blood away from the capillaries of the skin beds directly into small veins and thus back to the heart to help preserve the core temperature of the body when metabolism is so low that heat production is inadequate. In this way most of the blood flow to the hands and feet is cut off in many individuals who are hypothyroid. This is the reason so many hypothyroid individuals complain of having cold hands and feet. When this vaso-constriction in the hands is marked, the condition is called Raynaud's syndrome and can be a symptom of a number of different diseases.

Humans have used the same strategy the body uses for years to try to keep warm. If there is not enough heat to heat the whole house one or two rooms will be chosen to heat. Since heat is needed for cooking, the family will congregate in the kitchen until bedtime before going to the cold bedrooms to sleep.

The collection of mucin or polysaccharides responsible for the myxedema of hypothyroidism (which is described in the chapter on connective tissue disease) is felt to make the whole situation worse by some clinicians. They believe these polysaccharides which collect in hypothyroidism tend to collect around the small blood vessels which supply nutrients to the skin. The nutrients present in these capillaries have to pass through a mucous barrier before they can reach the cells that need them. Clinicians describe the situation as similar to wearing rubber gloves under the skin. Thus the skin is not able to get the needed nutrients and is left undernourished. This poor nutrition is aggravated by the fact that these polysaccharides hold tightly onto water. Edema is common which adds to the distance nutrients must travel to supply the skin.

Skin is a dynamic organ. The outer layers are constantly being shed and replaced every few days. Without proper nutrition the skin cannot be replaced adequately and it becomes susceptible to a whole variety of diseases. Even when outright rashes do not appear, hypothyroid patients have many complaints associated with skin. The commonest complaint is that the skin is dry. This dry skin is aggravated in the winter when scattered patches of dry skin occur, perhaps partly due to the fact that in winter the body has to expend extra energy just to keep up its core temperature. Soaps which tend to remove oil and moisture from the skin and increase its dryness must be used more cautiously during the winter months.

This skin dryness in turn may affect some of the sensory organs embedded in the skin, such as the nerve endings responding to touch, pain, heat, and cold. It is common for those who are hypothyroid to complain of strange sensations in the skin. A common sensation is compared to having ants crawling under the skin. In fact nearly eighty percent of hypothyroid patients will report some abnormal skin sensations if questioned closely.[76]

Other structures connected with the skin do not function in a normal way either. For example, hypothyroid patients often complain of problems with sweating---they either sweat too much, to the point of embarrassment, or not enough. If they sweat too much this, in turn, tends to aggravate a number of skin rashes. If they do not sweat enough, they have a hard time cooling their body down in the heat of summer. So they are intolerant to both heat and cold.

The fingernails are not adequately nourished and may grow extremely slowly. Brittleness and cracking of the nails is common. Diseases of the nails are much more frequent. The growth of hair is also affected. Hair in hypothyroidism loses its luster, becomes dry and coarse, and tends to fall out. Almost half of patients who are hypothyroid have significant concerns about their hair. There are some other interesting associations of hair with hypothyroidism. For some reason red hair seems to be a marker for hypothyroidism, and some clinicians believe that a majority of redheads are hypothyroid. Premature graying of the hair also has a very strong association with hypothyroidism.

The amount of pigment in the skin, thus the skin's color, may be affected by hypothyroidism. Some of these effects are direct, others are indirect. For example individuals who are low thyroid tend to be anemic because red cell production is slowed. Also since the blood flow to the skin is cut down, individuals tend to be pale since there is not as much red blood in the capillary beds nourishing the skin, thus there is less red pigment. This is a direct effect. An indirect effect is the fact that, in hypothyroidism, the liver has a hard time converting beta carotene to active vitamin A. So beta carotene builds up in the body giving the skin a lightly yellowish hue. One can see vitiligo, patches of skin without normal pigmentation in hypothyroidism. Though the cause is unknown, hypothyroidism makes this condition worse. Certain fungus infections of the skin mimic this condition giving the skin a patchy appearance as well.

In skin, type II de-iodinase is active in transforming T4 to the much more active T3 preparation. This transformation is greatly enhanced by glucocorticoids. Glucocorticoid skin preparations such as hydrocortisone are the mainstay in the treatment of a multitude of skin conditions. These preparations are actually increasing the levels of T3 in the skin. When strong cortisone preparations are used for

---

[76]Broda O. Barnes, Lawrence Galton; **Hypothyroidism the Unsuspected Illness**, Thomas Y Crowell Company, New York, 1976.

prolonged periods on the skin of the face, reactions occur which indicate the skin is being overstimulated. Small net-works of blood vessels appear to try to bring in the nutrients required by this skin that has become metabolically over-active. These blood vessels, once formed, may not go away and produce a particularly unsightly and unwanted blemish on the face. For this reason strong steroids are not to be used on the face for more than very short periods of time.

Minor skin problems and the growth problems involving nails and hair respond dramatically to thyroid replacement therapy. Hair usually stops falling out, loses its coarseness and becomes more lustrous. Fingernails start to grow again and strengthen. The skin softens in texture, and most rashes respond dramatically as well.

Both bacterial and fungus infections are common on the skin. Acne is the most common of these conditions. It is often greatly improved by being on thyroid. Cortisone is occasionally used by dermatologists to try to control severe cases. Boils usual will not occur unless an individual is hypothyroid, nor will other skin abscesses. Again, severe skin infections of any kind only seem to occur in individuals who are hypothyroid, as the skin lacks the nutrition and metabolism to fight those infections off.

Allergic skin reactions of all kinds respond to both thyroid and adrenal preparations. In milder problems, just thyroid will suffice. But if problems are more severe the glucocorticoids may need to be added. Thyroid by itself will clear about half of skin rashes. Many allergic rashes benefit by the addition of the cortisones. If a rash is severe, one may want to use both medications together from the beginning.

What is true of allergic rashes is also true of most other skin rashes. Certain skin conditions do not respond well to thyroid by itself. One of these conditions is psoriasis. Though occasionally psoriasis will clear just with thyroid replacement therapy, this is not usually the case. If a serious attempt is being made to control the psoriasis, either topical or oral steroids will probably be needed.

Hypothyroidism affects the whole outward appearance of the body. Thyroid therapy will often give an appearance of renewed vitality. And this renewed vitality will be more than skin deep.

Conclusion

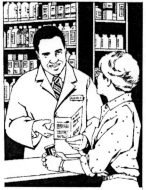

Many more illustrations on the effect of thyroid on an individual's health could be given. If symptoms are severe, each patient has a dramatic story to tell on how much difference taking thyroid, along with adrenal support when needed, has made.

Many doctors down through the years have tried to call attention to the importance of hypothyroidism in such books as *Hypothyroidism, the Unsuspected Illness* and *The Miracle of Feeling Well.* Perhaps this book will help accomplish what the other books have failed to do: make the medical profession truly aware of the importance of unrecognized hypothyroidism.

The fact is that every part of the body is touched by thyroid hormone. So true health is not possible if thyroid function is deficient. Unfortunately the medical profession has concentrated on the control mechanism that keeps the blood levels of thyroid hormone on an even keel. Most of them have ignored a second control mechanism in the cells themselves that controls the intercellular activity of thyroid hormone, the balance of T3, RT3 and T4 in the cells, which for most individuals is far more important. Unless the T3 levels are adequate, patients are functionally hypothyroid. Thyroid is one of the three key legs which provide the energy, the power for the body to perform its tasks---everything from thinking, to physical activities, to running myriads of chemical processes. The other two legs of the triad are nutrition, which provides the basic ingredients the body needs, and the adrenal system which regulates the supplies. The thyroid provides the control.

Our bodies need to be tuned to the greatest possible efficiency to cope with the increase in chronic disease, and with the increase in environmental challenges in our shrinking world. Making sure that your thyroid gland is functioning properly is a way of guaranteeing that your body is up to the health challenges it may face.

Perhaps you are one of the many who have a metabolism that is sluggish and are lacking in T3 at a cellular level. If you are, thyroid replacement therapy could make a dramatic difference in your life, could stop or slow down any deteriorating health you have and could restore you to a renewed level of vitality.

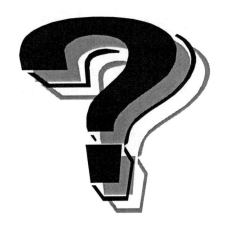

Speculations on Thyroid Function

Though much is known about the functioning of thyroid hormone even more aspects remain a mystery. One mysterious area is the functioning of Type I de-iodinase. It appears that Type I de-iodinase controls both the conversion of T4 to T3 and RT3. What shifts the amount of T3 versus RT3 produced under the influence of Type I de-iodinase is not known. RT3 acts as a competitive inhibitor--- blocks the activity of T3. I suspect that the pH within the cells is critical, with a more alkaline pH favoring the formation of T3. Exercise, with anaerobic energy production, increases the acidity in the cells. This, I suspect, is a limiting mechanism which prevents metabolism from running out of control. It is known that a diet which shifts the pH towards the alkaline side, increases energy, increases metabolism, so it is logical that more T3 is being produced. It is also known that athletes tend to be low thyroid. All their aerobic exercise with the production of lactic acid apparently slows metabolism. The slow heart rates of those in "good condition" is one evidence of this. Certain deep breathing exercises which blow off CO_2 cause a respiratory alkalosis and also seems to increases the rate of metabolism. I know of no research on the subject..

Much of the interplay between thyroid and the various adrenal hormone also is little researched and little understood. In the brain prednisone greatly enhances the production of T3. The adrenal hormones pregnenolone, DHEA and estrogen all sharpen functions of the brain such as memory. Estrogen also gives some protection against Alzheimer's. Does estrogen's ability to bind to thyroid binding sites in the brain play a role in this protection and mental sharpening? Or is the production of T3 increased? Since both T3 and 3 omega fatty acids improve depression do these entities complement each other in some way? These questions might provide fruitful areas for research. The questions are endless and the answers may lead to a better answer to many mental miseries.

Both brain development and skeletal development take place rapidly in the newborn with adrenal and thyroid hormone levels that are sky high as compared to an adult. If both thyroid and adrenal hormones are increased in an adult in balanced fashion, would the healing time for fractures be reduced? Would the body be able to reverse brain damage after strokes or paralysis after spinal cord injury? It is known that Pregnenolone by itself is helpful in spinal cord injuries.

The fact that thyroid hormone not only works in the nucleus of cells but also directly in the mitochondria is recent information. Perhaps, the structure of thyroid hormone allows roles that have not been suspected in the past. Though it is not included in the lists of the amino acids the body uses to build protein, structurally it is an amino acid and should be able to attach to all proteins. It is now known that thyroid hormone is active while bound to other protein molecules. What significance could this binding have? It seems to enhance thyroid function in some experiments.

The oldest method of measuring thyroid function was the basal metabolism. It was measured by measuring the oxygen consumption of the body. It is known that electro-magnetic fields can be used to increase oxygen consumption. Does the electro-magnetic field increase thyroid function in some way? That question should be explored. It is possible that thyroid is able to pick up electro-magnetic signals and transmits that energy in some fashion which increases metabolism. If thyroid is indeed sensitive to electro-magnetic energy, exercise which increases blood flow could immediately signal the body to increase its metabolism. How could it do so? Charged particles, ions are present in the blood. Moving charged particles generates magnetic fields. Increasing the speed of these charged particles, will increase the strength of the magnetic field, possibly signally this information to thyroid hormone. Since the body's energy needs fluctuate, tying metabolism to the electro-magnetic field should provide a system that is very sensitive to changing metabolic needs. Again there is no research in this area. Further research will undoubtably eventually revolutionize our understanding of thyroid function.

But if just what is known about thyroid function is taught and applied by the medical profession, tremendous progress would be made in the treatment of degenerative disease. The control of thyroid function is so complex and so fundamental to the functioning of the body that when better understood will revolutionize medicine's approach to many diseases in which the relationship to hypothyroidism is not presently suspected.

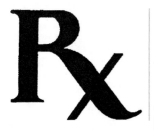

GLOSSARY

Atom---The smallest unit of an element.

ACTH (adrenocortocotropic hormone)---A hormone secreted by the anterior pituitary gland. It stimulates the adrenal gland to make steroids.

Amino acid---The basic structural unit of proteins. Twenty-two different amino acids are used by the body to form all proteins. Eight of these are called essential because the body is not able to manufacture them. They must be provided by food or supplements.

Antibody---A protein produced by the body to neutralize or destroy an antigen.

Antigen---A substance usually foreign to the body such as a bacteria, virus, or toxin to which the body reacts by forming antibodies.

Atrial fibrillation---Irregular, often very rapid beating of the heart due to rapid rate of impulses coming from the pacemaker in the atria or upper chamber of the heart.

Autoimmune---Immunity refers to the ability to fight off diseases. In autoimmune conditions, the body is fighting against itself.

Autonomic nervous system---The nervous system that controls normal, unconscious body functions.

Cell membrane--The outer layer of the cell, largely made up of fatty acids.

Cholesterol---A fat-like substance which is the precursor of all the active steroids in the body. Two thirds of the cholesterol in the body is manufactured by the liver, so dietary control of cholesterol is somewhat limited.

Desiccated---To dry out thoroughly. In medicine it frequently refers to glandular products which have had their water content removed, usually through a process of vacuum extraction, so heat is not used, thus preserving the activity of the hormone.

DHEA---An adrenal hormone which declines with age. It has important functions relating to the memory and to the immune system.

Ecchinoids---Cellular hormones manufactured from essential fatty acids.

Element---A substance made up of atoms having the same number of protons in their nucleus.

Estrogen---A hormone made both by the adrenal glands and ovaries. It can also be produced by fat cells. Estrogen promotes female characteristics but is also found in smaller amounts in males.   The estrogens manufactured by the body are estrone, estradiol, and estriol.

Glandular---Crude extract of tissue from a gland such as the adrenal or thymus.

Glucocorticoids---Steroid compounds capable of significantly influencing carbohydrate metabolism. They promote glycogen deposition in the liver, release of lipids from fat stores and the production of glucose from protein. They also have marked anti-inflammatory effects.

Glucagon---A hormone produced by the pancreas which releases glucose from body stores thus increasing blood sugar.

HAIT: Hashimoto's Thyroiditis---Common autoimmune disease of the thyroid gland which gradually destroys thyroid tissue

Hormone---A chemical messenger which is produced by a gland and has major metabolic effects on other parts of the body.

Homocystein---Breakdown product of the amino acid Cystein which is very irritating to blood vessels.

Hydrocortisone---Major glucocorticoid produced by the body. This steroid is frequently used to treat skin diseases.

Hypothalamus---A small area near the base of the brain, above and behind the roof of the mouth which is an important control center for many hormones, monitoring their levels in the body.

Insulin---A hormone made by the beta cells of the pancreas which helps sugar enter cells thus, helping control blood sugar levels.

Libido: The sex drive

Metabolism---The chemical processes continuously going on in the body involving the production of energy and/or the breakdown or creation of new molecules.

Mineral corticoids: Steroids which regulate mineral and water balance.

Mitochondria---power plant of the cells where glucose is converted to energy.

Molecule---The smallest possible quantity of atoms that retain the chemical properties of the substance in question.

Neuron---A brain cell. There are over 100 billion of these cells in the brain which are connected to a multitude of other neurons. Neurons communicate with each other through neurotransmitters.

Neurotransmitter---A biochemical substance that relays messages from one neuron to another.   Norepinephrine,   serotonin,   and   dopamine   are   common neurotransmitters.

Norepinephrine---A hormone made by the adrenal medulla similar to epinephrine, part of the autonomic nervous system..

Pituitary Gland---Gland at the base of the brain which produces ACTH, which controls the adrenal gland, and TSH, which controls the thyroid gland

Precursor---A substance that precedes and is the source or building block of another substance.

Prednisone---Synthetic glucocorticoid which is roughly 4 times stronger than hydrocortisone. Its advantage is that it is taken one time a day rather than 4 times. It is converted to its active form in the liver and so it does not cause as much suppression of the adrenal gland.

Pregnenolone: The first of the adrenal hormones, precursor of all other adrenal hormones. It is active in its own right, improving short term memory, for example.

Progesterone---A hormone produced by the ovaries and the adrenal gland which counters certain properties of estrogen.   It prepares the uterine lining, the endometrium, for the implantation of a fertilized egg.

Prostaglandins: Any of a group of physiologically active hormone-like substances obtained from essential fatty acids. They occur in various human body tissues affecting blood pressure, metabolism and smooth muscle activity.

Receptor---A special arrangement of cells that allows another molecule such as a hormone to interact, often stimulating the cell in a specific way.

Testosterone---A hormone made by the testicles and adrenal glands that promotes masculine traits.

Thyroid---Iodine-containing hormone of the thyroid gland which regulates the metabolism of the body.

T4----Thyroxine, the thyroid hormone which contains four iodine atoms and is the transport form of thyroid. Ninety-five % of thyroid measured in the bloodstream is in the form of T4.

T3---Liothyronine, thyroid hormone containing three iodine atoms which is responsible for most of the metabolism which takes place in the cell.

TRH: Thyrotropin Releasing Hormone is a tri-peptide (contains three amino acids) which stimulates the release of TSH from the anterior pituitary and also functions as a neurotransmitter.

TSH: Hormone produced by the anterior pituitary which controls the release of thyroid hormones from the thyroid gland.

ISBN 1553696131

9 781553 696131